中医五 病机

Pathomechanisms of the

Zhōng Yī Wǔ Zàng Bìng Jī Xué

肺病之病機

Pathomechanisms of the LUNG

Fèi Bìng Zhī Bìng Jī

Yán Shí-Lín, Lǐ Zhèng-Huá

Edited by Nigel Wiseman and Anthony Venuti
Translated by Sabine Wilms

Paradigm Publications
Taos, New Mexico 2011

Pathomechanisms of the Five Viscera

Volume Four

Pathomechanisms of the Lung

Yán Shí Lín 严石林 Lǐ Zhèng-Huá 李正华

Translated by Sabine Wilms

Edited by Nigel Wiseman and Anthony Venuti

202 Bendix Drive, Taos, New Mexico 87571 USA

www.paradigm-pubs.com

Distributed by Redwing Book Company

www.redwingbooks.com

COMP Designation: Original Chinese work in English translation

Library of Congress Cataloging-in-Publication Data

Yan, Shi Lin, 1943-
[Zhong Yi Wu Zang Bing Ji Xue: Xin Bing Zhi Bing Ji. English]
Pathomechanisms of the five viscera: pathomechanisms of the heart / Yan Shi Lin, Li Zheng-Hua ; with
the assistance of Yan Yan ... [et al.] ; translated by Wang Ying and Sabine Wilms ; edited by Eric Brand and Zhang Yu Huan.
p. ; cm.
Includes bibliographical references and index.
ISBN 0-912111-79-8
1. Heart--Pathophysiology. 2. Medicine, Chinese. I. Li, Zheng-Hua,
1942- . II. Brand, Eric, 1978- . III. Wiseman, Nigel. IV. Title.
[DNLM: 1. Heart--physiopathology. 2. Medicine, Chinese Traditional.
WG 200 Y21z 2005a]
RC682.9.Y36125 2005
616.1'2--dc22

2005023189

Library of Congress Number: 2005023189

International Standard Book Number (ISBN-13): 978091211872

Printed in the United States of America

Table of Contents

Introduction

Pathomechanisms of the Lung

The lung is located above the diaphragm in the center of the chest. Its position is the highest and it is shaped like a canopy for the five viscera and six bowels, and thus is called the "florid canopy." The lobes of the lung are delicate; when vacuous, they resemble a bee's nest and cannot bear cold or heat. Its nature is to depurate. The "Treatise on the Twelve Offices in the *Nèi Jīng* ("The Inner Canon")" in the *Yī Guàn* ("Thorough Knowledge of Medicine") explains:

> "Below the throat is the lung. Its two lobes are white and glisten like jade. It is called the florid canopy and it covers all the viscera. It is empty and resembles a bee's nest, with no outlet for qì at the bottom. Therefore it is full upon inhalation and empty upon exhalation."

The lung has the physiological functions of governing qì, managing breathing, regulating the waterways, diffusing defense qì, and assembling the hundred vessels. It also governs management and regulation, the skin and body hair, and the sense of smell and production of sounds. Because of the lung's location, structure, and functional peculiarities, lung disease tends to manifests in the following pathomechanical changes.

肺病病机

肺位于膈上，居于胸中，位置最高，形盖五脏六腑，故有“华盖”之称。肺叶娇嫩，虚如蜂窠，不耐寒热，其性清肃。如《医贯•内经十二官论》说：“喉下为肺，两叶白莹，谓之华盖，以复诸脏。虚如蜂巢，下无透气，故吸之则满，呼之则虚。”肺有主气、司呼吸，通调水道，宣散卫气，朝百脉、主治节，主皮毛，主嗅觉和发声等生理功能。肺脏自身的位置结构和功能特点，使肺发病之后，常呈现下列病机变化。

Irregularities in the breathing function: The lung governs breathing and is the place where qì from inside the body is exchanged with gases from the outside. When disease evil invades the lung, the respiratory movements become abnormal. This can easily manifest in inhibited breathing or dyspnea. In severe cases, it can lead to respiratory failure.

呼吸功能失调：肺主呼吸，是体内外气体的交换场所。病邪犯肺，呼吸运动异常，易见呼吸不畅、呼吸困难等表现，甚者可引起呼吸功能衰竭。

Abnormalities in the function of governing qì: The lung governs all qì. It is closely linked to the generation of qì and the upbearing, downbearing, and inward and outward movement of the qì dynamic. When disease occurs in the lung, it is unable to perfuse the upper orifices. This can lead to stoppage in the upper orifices and inhibited breathing. When it is unable to depurate and downbear lung qì, this can prevent liver qì from downbearing and cause it to rebel counterflow against lung-metal. It can also cause stomach qì to ascend counterflow, resulting in stoppage of bowel qì. Lastly, it can prevent the kidney from absorbing qì, so that qì fails to return to its origin. If the lung is unable to diffuse defense qì, it can lead to insecurity of the defensive exterior. If it is unable to transform and engender ancestral qì, it can debilitate visceral qì and lower functions in the whole body.

主气功能异常：肺主诸气，与气的生成和气机升降出入运动有密切关系。肺发病时，不能宣通上窍，可致上窍不通，呼吸不利。不能肃降肺气，可致肝气不降，逆侮肺金；胃气上逆，腑气不通；肾气不纳，气不归元。不能宣发卫气，可致卫表不固。不能化生宗气，可使脏气衰微，全身功能低下。

Irregularities in the fluid metabolism: The lung governs regulation of the waterways and is the upper source of water. It is closely linked to the distribution and elimination of fluids. Failure of the lung to distribute liquid can cause loss of nourishment in the internal organs and the orifices. When qì fails to transform liquid, water-humor collects. This can engender dampness, which transforms into rheum and phlegm. When qì fails to move water, water qì floods. This can cause generalized water swelling. When the lung is vacuous and loses control, the fluids are not distributed, but rush straight into the lower body. This can lead to enuresis, urinary frequency, and long voidings of clear urine.

津液代谢失调：肺主通调水道，为水之上源，与津液的输布、排泄密切相关。肺不布津，可使脏腑形体官窍失于滋养；气不化津，水液停聚，可生湿成饮化痰；气不行水，水气泛溢，可致全身水肿；肺虚失制，水津不布，直趋于下，可致遗尿、小便频数、清长。

Inhibited blood movement: The lung assembles the hundred vessels. Ancestral qì has the function of passing through the heart vessel and moving qì and blood. When the lung is diseased and therefore unable to assist the heart in moving blood, the heart and lung share the disease. This can lead to stasis and obstruction in the blood flow.

血液运行不畅：肺朝百脉，宗气有贯心脉而行气血的作用。肺病不能助心行血，心肺同病，可致血行瘀阻。

Insecurity of the external defense function: The lung governs the skin and body hair; it serves as a protective screen against external evil. When external evil invades and entraps defense qì, lung qì suffers encumbrance. This can easily engender the pathological change of lung defense failing to diffuse.

卫外功能不固：肺主皮毛，为防御外邪的屏障。外邪侵袭，卫气被遏，肺气受困，故易发生肺卫失宣的病变。

Summary of Pathomechanisms of the Lung

1. Irregularities in Breathing
    - Inhibited breathing, dyspnea.
2. Abnormalities in Regulating Qì
    - Loss of diffusion in the upper orifices: Block in the orifices.
    - Irregularities in depurative downbearing:
        - Liver qì failing to downbear: Counterflow rebellion against lung-metal.
        - Counterflow ascent of stomach qì: Stoppage of bowel qì.
        - Kidney failing to perform qì transformation: Qì failing to return to its origin.
        - Non-engenderment of ancestral qì: Debilitation of visceral qì.
3. Fluid Disorder
    - Lung failing to distribute the fluids: Loss of enrichment in the orifices.
    - Qì failing to transform liquid: Collection of water-humor, engenderment of dampness transforming into rheum and phlegm.
    - Qì failing to move water: Water qì spillage, water swelling.
    - Lung vacuity and loss of control: Enuresis, urinary frequency, long voidings of clear urine.
4. Failure to Move Blood
    - Stasis and obstruction of the blood flow.
5. Insecurity of External Defense
    - Lung defense failing to diffuse.

肺病病机

1. 呼吸失调: 呼吸不畅，呼吸困难。

2. 主气失常:

  上窍失宣: 官窍闭塞。

  肃降失调:

    肝气不降: 逆侮肺金。

    胃气上逆: 腑气不通。

    肾气不化: 气不归元。

    宗气不生: 脏气衰微。

3. 津液失调:

    肺不布津: 官窍失滋。

    气不化津: 水液停聚、生湿化饮成痰。

    气不行水: 水气泛溢、水肿。

    肺虚失制: 遗尿、尿频、小便清长。

4. 血液不运: 血行瘀阻。

5. 卫外不固: 肺卫失宣。

1.1 Causes of Lung Disease

Lung disease can be due to a number of different causes. External contraction of the six excesses impairs diffusion and downbearing of the lung. Dietary irregularities cause phlegm-rheum to collect internally. Affect-mind disharmony depresses and damages the lung. An invasion of consumption "worms" depletes qì and yīn. Injury from taxation fatigue causes insufficiency of right qì. In addition, constitutional insufficiency, weak health in old age, enduring or severe disease, lack of or inappropriate treatment, and shifts from other diseases can all lead to pathomechanical changes in the lung.

Pathological changes in the lung are extremely complex. Nevertheless, we can summarily state that the most basic changes are breakdown of qì transformation and obstruction of fluid metabolism. These manifest as pathological trends toward qì and liquid disorders. At the same time, the lung is able to perform its many physiological functions only as a result of its activities of diffusing and depurative downbearing. For this reason, lung disease commonly hinges on disorders of diffusing and depurative downbearing.

The concepts of lung repletion and lung vacuity have been recognized ever since the *Huáng Dì Nèi Jīng* ("The Yellow Emperor's Inner Canon"). The "General Treatise on Vacuity and Repletion" in the *Sù Wèn* ("Plain Questions") explained: "Qì vacuity means lung vacuity." The treatise on "Methods of Treating Visceral Qì in Accordance with the Seasons" in the same text stated: "Lung disease manifests in qì counterflow panting and cough, and shoulder and back pain… Vacuity results in shortage of qì with inability to catch one's breath, deafness, and dry throat." The "Treatise on Major Strange Diseases" of the same text also included the theory that lung fullness always means repletion: "Liver fullness, kidney fullness, and lung fullness all refer to repletion and precisely mean swelling. In the case of the lung, it means congestion, panting, and fullness in both subaxillary regions." The chapter, "Root Spirit" in the *Líng Shū* ("The Magic Pivot") further pointed out: "The lung stores qì… and when it is replete, it causes panting with a howling sound, fullness in the chest, and breathing while looking upward." This was the first classification of lung disease into the pathomechanisms of vacuity and repletion.

Most medical classics and formularies in later ages have also discussed the pathomechanisms of lung disease under the principle of vacuity and repletion. Depending on differences in the disease cause, external contraction of the six excesses, internal damage by the seven affects, internal lodging of pathologic substances, fierce struggle between right and evil, severe pathologic activity, and exuberance and superabundance mostly manifest in pathomechanisms that tend toward repletion. On the other hand, an excessive exuberance of evil qì or an excessively prolonged disease condition can damage right qì. When the qì and blood and yīn and yáng in the lung are insufficient, organ functions and activities are weakened and decline. This reflects pathomechanical changes that tend toward vacuity.

肺病的病因

外感六淫，肺失宣降；饮食不节，痰饮内停；情志失调，抑郁伤肺；痨虫侵袭，气阴亏损；劳倦损伤，正气不足；以及禀赋不足，年高体弱，久病重病，失治误治，其它疾病的传变，均可引起肺的病变。

肺的病理变化虽然十分复杂，然而归纳而言，最基本的变化却是气化失司和津液代谢障碍，表现为气津失调的病变趋向。同时由于肺的许多生理的功能都是通过肺的宣发和肃降两种运动形式而得以实现，故肺病常以宣发和肃降失调为机要。

从《黄帝内经》开始就有肺实和肺虚的提法，如《素问•通评虚实论》说："气虚者肺虚也。"《素问•脏气法时论》云："肺病者，喘咳逆气、肩背痛…。虚则少气不能报息，耳聋嗌干"。《素问•大奇论》有肺满皆实之说，"肝满肾满肺满皆实，即为肿。肺之壅喘而两胠满。"《灵枢•本神》进一步指出"肺藏气，…实则喘喝胸盈仰息。"成为肺病按虚、实病机分类之肇始。后世许多经典医著和方书，均以虚实为纲讨论肺病病机。根据致病原因的不同，外感六淫，内伤七情，病理产物停留，邪正剧烈相争，病理活动剧烈、亢盛有余，多表现出偏实为病机；邪气太盛，或病情迁延，正气受损，肺的气血阴阳不足，脏腑功能活动减弱、衰退降低，又反映出偏虚的病机变化。

Literature Review of Pathomechanisms of the Lung

📖 *Zá Bìng Yuán Liú Xī Zhú* ("Incisive Light on the Source of Miscellaneous Disease"), "The Origin and Development of Lung Disease"

> "The lung governs qì. It connects to the throat above and frees the orifices of the heart and liver below. It is in charge of the inward and outward movement of breath. It presides over the upper body by settling the various orifices, while also exerting pressure on the body's waste matter to move it to the large intestine. It discharges and absorbs clear qì. That which receives is yīn within greater yáng, in order to secure yáng qì; that which is in charge is yáng within greater yīn, in order to move yīn substances."

This quotation describes the important physiological functions of the lung: it governs qì, is in charge of breathing, and stands in an exterior-interior relationship with the large intestine.

📖 *Lín Zhèng Zhǐ Nán Yī Àn* ("A Clinical Guide with Case Histories"), "Lung Impediment"

> "The lung is the bellows of the breath. It is located highest up in the position of the sovereign, and it receives clear qì that is presented upward by the viscera and bowels. It is endowed with the ability to depurate, and its nature is to govern downbearing. But it is also the delicate viscus and cannot bear invasion by evil. In all cases, as soon as cold or the qì of the six excesses touch it, it can lead to disease. Its nature is averse to cold,

heat, and dryness, and it most fears wind-fire. When touched by evil, it loses its ability to depurate and downbear. As a consequence, congestion and stoppage arise."

This quotation expounds on how the lung, as the delicate viscus, by its nature governs depurative downbearing, but is easily invaded by the evil qì of the six excesses and loses its ability to depurate, which is an important pathomechanism.

🕮 *Zhōng Zàng Jīng* ("Central Treasury Canon"), "Discussing the Pulses and Patterns of Vacuity and Repletion, Cold and Heat, Life and Death, and Favorable and Unfavorable Shifts in Lung Disease"

"Vacuity, repletion, cold, and heat all make a person cough. Repletion results in dreams of weapons and of fear, as well as in raised-shoulder breathing and fullness in the chest. Vacuity results in cold, breathing with coughing, disinhibition in the lower body, shortage of qì and bodily strength, and increased sensation of sorrow."

This is a rather early text to put forth the notion of using vacuity and repletion as guiding principles for differentiating the pathomechanisms and clinical manifestations of lung disease.

🕮 *Zhū Bìng Yuán Hòu Lùn* ("The Origin and Indicators of Disease"), "Symptoms of Cough and Qì Ascent"

"Cough and qì ascent mean a superabundance of lung qì. When the lung contracts cold, in mild cases it causes coughing. The lung governs qì; when qì is superabundant, the result is panting and cough with qì ascent. This means that evil has struck qì so that qì becomes congested and cannot be diffused. A superabundance results, which is precisely the cause of cough and qì ascent. This condition is characterized by panting and cough with qì ascent, increased snivel and spittle, puffy swelling in the face and eyes, and qì counterflow."

This quotation discusses in detail the pathomechanical changes and manifestations of lung repletion, which are caused by evil qì invading the lung and by a superabundance of lung qì.

🕮 *Qiān Jīn Yào Fāng* ("A Thousand Gold Pieces Prescriptions"), "The Lung"

"The lung stores qì, which houses the corporeal soul. With regard to qì, it is associated with cough, and among the humors, with snivel. When lung qì is vacuous, it manifests in uninhibited and scant breathing through the nose, and when qì is replete, in dreams of warfare. When lung qì is exuberant, it manifests in dreams of fear and crying, and if reverse qì settles in the lung, in dreams of flying and visions of metal and iron implements."

This quotation indicates the different pathomechanical changes and manifestations that can result from lung qì vacuity and repletion.

📖 *Shèng Jì Zǒng Lù* ("Sages' Salvation Records"), "Section on the Lung Viscus"

> "[Lung] disease can arise from excess, which causes superabundance and results in a disease of superabundance. Deficiency, on the other hand, causes insufficiency, which also results in disease. Conditions of superabundance are referred to as lung repletion; conditions of insufficiency are referred to as lung vacuity. The symptoms of lung repletion are panting, cough, qì ascent, shoulder and back pain, sweating, and pain in the groin, knee, and lower leg. The symptoms of lung vacuity are coldness and pain in the shoulder and back, shortage of qì and inability to sigh deeply, fullness in the chest, and dry throat."

This is a more advanced description of the pathomechanisms and manifestations of lung vacuity and repletion on the basis of superabundance and deficiency.

📖 *Tú Shū Jí* ("Compendium of Books"), "Explanation of the Lung Viscus"

> "When a person's body is yellowish black, it indicates debilitation of lung qì. When a person presents with increased sound, it indicates lung exuberance. When a person is unable to endure cold, it indicates lung debilitation. When a person loves to eat acrid foods, it indicates an insufficiency of lung qì. When a person's intestines rumble, it indicates lung congestion."

From the angle of sound, complexion, likes, and dislikes, this quotation illustrates the pathomechanical changes and manifestations of lung qì vacuity and repletion.

📖 *Yī Xué Rù Mén* ("The Gateway to Medicine"), "The Internal Organs"

> "Qì counterflow with glomus in the chest and back pain mean panting, wheezing, and huffing. When lung qì is excessive, it causes panting and cough, qì counterflow, back pain, an angry manner, and possibly fullness and oppression of the qì dynamic in the chest and diaphragm, stretching into back pain ... When heat affects the lung, it causes pain in the throat, diaphragm, sacrum and coccyx, groin, and knees, as well as drinker's nose and nose piles, possibly forming abscesses. The lung penetrates to the throat and tongue; its state is reflected in the center of the chest. Therefore heat congestion results in swelling and pain in the throat and tongue, fullness and oppression in the chest and diaphragm, and pain in the sacrum and coccyx, groin, and knees. When this causes crippling wilt, it means lung heat scorching the lobes... Extreme vacuity manifests in faint breathing during inhalation and exhalation, yawning and stretching, urinary frequency, and in lung wilting and welling-abscess, possibly

> forming consumption. The lung governs qì; when it is vacuous, it manifests in breathing with shortage of qì, insufficient respiration, and urinary frequency or enuresis. When the vacuity is severe, it is exploited by the ministerial fire. This results in bloody cough, possibly to the point of consumption, welling-abscess of the lung, and lung wilting."

This is a fairly comprehensive description of the pathomechanisms of lung repletion and lung vacuity, as well as of the resulting disease patterns and clinical manifestations.

文献评述

《杂病源流犀烛•肺病源流》曰"肺主气，上连咽喉，下通心肝之窍，司呼吸出入，君上以镇诸窍，而压糟粕，以行于大肠。出纳清气，所受者太阳之阴，以固阳气。所司者太阴之阳，以行阴物。"阐述了肺有主气，司呼吸，与大肠互为表里的重要生理功能。

《临证指南医案•肺痹》曰: "肺为呼吸之橐龠，位君最高，受脏腑上朝之清气，禀清肃之体，性主乎降，又为娇脏，不耐邪侵，凡冷六淫之气，一有所著，即能致病。其性恶寒，恶热，恶燥，最畏风火。邪著则失清肃降令，遂痹塞不通爽矣。"阐述肺为娇脏，性主肃降，易被六淫邪气侵犯，失其清肃，引起发病的重要病机。

《中藏经•论肺脏虚实寒热生死逆顺脉证之法》曰: "虚实寒热皆使人咳嗽。实则梦刀兵恐惧，肩息胸满。虚则寒生咳息利下，少气力，多悲感。"较早提出以虚实为纲分辨肺病病机及临床表现。

《诸病源候论•咳嗽上气候》曰: "夫咳嗽上气者，肺气有余也。肺感于寒，微者则成咳嗽。肺主气，气有余则喘咳上气，此为邪搏于气，气壅不得宣发，是为有余，故咳嗽而上气也。其状喘咳上气，多涕唾而面目胕 肿气逆也。" 详细论述邪气犯肺，肺气有余而致肺实的病机变化及表现。

《千金要方•肺脏》曰: "肺藏气，气舍魄，在气为咳，在液为涕。肺气虚，则鼻息利少，气实，则梦见兵战; 肺气盛，则梦恐惧哭泣; 厥气客于肺，则梦飞扬，见金铁之器物。"指出肺气虚实可引起性质不同的病机变化及表现。

《圣济总录•肺脏门》曰: "病所由生，过为有余，有余病也。不及为不足，不足亦病也。有余之病，是谓肺实。不足之病，是谓肺虚。肺实之证，喘嗽上气，肩背痛汗出，阴股膝胫皆痛是也。肺虚之证，肩背寒痛，少气不能太息，胸满嗌干是也。"进一步从有余不足讨论肺病虚实的病机及表现。

《图书编•肺脏说》曰: ，“人之体黧者，肺气衰也。人之多声音者，肺之盛也。人之不耐寒者，肺衰也。人者好食辛者，肺气不足也。人之肠鸣者，肺壅也。”从声色喜恶方面阐明肺气虚实的病机变化及表现。

《医学入门•脏腑》曰: “气逆胸痞背痛, 喘哮息本膹. 肺气太过则令人喘咳, 气逆, 背痛, 愠愠然, 或胸膈膹闷之, 气牵引背疼…热著, 咽膈尻阴股膝皆痛, 鼻鼽、鼻痔、或成渊. 肺通喉舌, 候在胸中, 故热壅则喉舌肿痛, 胸膈满闷, 尻阴股膝痛为痿躄者, 肺热叶焦也…虚极, 呼吸息微, 欠伸溺频, 肺痿、肺痈、或成瘵. 肺主气, 虚则呼吸少气, 不足以息, 小便频数, 或遗. 虚甚为相火所乘, 则咳而见血, 或为痨瘵、肺痈、肺痿. ” 较为全面论述肺实肺虚的病机变化和引起的各种病证及临床表现.

Part One

Pathomechanisms of Lung Repletion

Introduction

Lung Repletion

The *Huáng Dì Nèi Jīng* ("The Yellow Emperor's Inner Canon") already mentioned the phrase "lung qì exuberance" and discussed the changes related to this pathomechanism from the perspective of pulse signs. For example, the "Treatise on Morbid Bearing" in the *Sù Wèn* ("Plain Questions") states: "When lung qì is exuberant, the pulse is large; when the pulse is large, the patient is unable to lie flat." The chapter "On Diseases Caused by Excesses and Evils" in the *Líng Shū* ("The Magic Pivot") contains the following description: "When lung qì is exuberant, it causes dreams of fear, of crying, and of flying upward." This indicates that lung qì exuberance can lead to abnormalities of the essence-spirit. From this, we can see that the *Nèi Jīng* ("The Inner Canon") already rudimentarily described the pathomechanism of lung repletion.

However, it is mentioned more concretely in the *Zhōng Zàng Jīng* ("Central Treasury Canon"). Categorizing lung pathomechanisms into vacuity and repletion, this book contains a separate chapter, "Discussion of the Pulses and Patterns of Vacuity and Repletion, Cold and Heat, Life and Death, and Favorable and Unfavorable Shifts in the Lung." In addition, it specifically mentions the term "lung repletion disease" and synthesizes the types and pulse patterns of the pathomechanism of lung repletion. It explains that "Lung repletion disease results in qì ascent, rapid panting, cough, generalized heat effusion, and a large pulse."

Slightly later, the chapter, "Symptoms of Lung Disease" in the *Zhū Bìng Yuán Hòu Lùn* ("The Origin and Indicators of Disease") also explained:

> "When lung qì is exuberant, it means that qì is superabundant. This results in panting and cough with qì ascent, shoulder and back pain, sweating, and pain in the sacrum and coccyx, groin, lower leg, and foot. All these indicate a repletion of lung qì."

This text pointed out that lung qì exuberance results in the pathomechanism of lung qì repletion. Subsequently, the *Qiān Jīn Yào Fāng* ("A Thousand Gold Pieces Prescriptions"), *Shèng Jì Zǒng Lù* ("Sages' Salvation Records"), and *Yán Shì Jì Shēng Fāng* ("Yan's Remedies for Curing All People") discussed the pathomechanism and manifestations of lung repletion in even greater depth.

Observations in clinical practice indicate that in a majority of cases, disease in the lung tends towards a pathomechanism of repletion. This is primarily related to the activity of diffusing and depurative downbearing by the lung. When evil qì of the six excesses assails the body from the mouth and nose or through the skin and body hair, it rouses lung defense qì to fight against evil. Right and evil struggle with each other, and evil qì is repressed. At the same time, however, the diffusing movement of the lung is impeded, defense qì is trapped, and lung qì is encumbered. This creates the pathomechanism of dual repletion of lung and defense.

Disease evil can pass from the exterior to the interior and invade the center of the lung; alternatively, pathologic substances can arise internally and collect in the center of the lung. Regardless of whether it is a case of cold evil congealing and stagnating or of heat evil dispersing and scorching, the congestion of phlegm-rheum and water-damp can equally obstruct lung qì and disorder diffusing and depurative downbearing. This gives rise to a host of pathomechanical changes that are related to evil qì hyperactivity and exuberance, and to disease conditions tending towards repletion.

Because the key manifestations of lung repletion are disturbances of diffusion and downbearing, the pathomechanism of lung repletion includes three aspects: impaired diffusion of the lung; impaired depurative downbearing of the lung; and impaired diffusion and downbearing of the lung.

肺实的病机

《黄帝内经》中已开始有“肺气盛”的提法，并从脉症方面讨论肺气盛的病机变化。如《素问•病能》有：“肺气盛则脉大，脉大则不能偃卧。”《灵枢•淫邪发病篇》有：“肺气盛，则梦恐惧，哭泣，飞扬”等论述，指出肺气盛可引起精神失调。可以看出《内经》已初步提到肺实的病机。但最为明确提出肺实病机的应是《中藏经》，此书不仅把肺的病机按虚、实分类，有《论肺脏虚实寒热生死逆顺脉证之法》的专章，而且直接点出“肺实病”的名称，综合肺实病机的典型脉症说：“肺实病则上气喘急咳嗽，身热脉大也。”随之《诸病源候论•肺病候》也说：“肺气盛，为气有余，则也。”随之《诸病源候论•肺病候》也说:“肺气盛，为气有余，则病喘咳上气，肩背痛，汗出，尻阴股胫足皆痛，是为肺气之实也。”肯定了肺气盛则为肺气实之病机。其后，《千金要方》、《圣济总录》《济生方》更深入探讨了肺实的病机和表现。临床实践观察表明，肺脏发病时，病机偏实者居多。其原因主要与肺的宣发、肃降运动有关。六淫邪气从口鼻、皮毛侵袭人体，肺卫之气奋起抗邪，邪正相争，邪气受抑，同时肺的宣发运动亦受阻碍，卫气被遏，肺气被困，形成肺卫俱实的病机。若病邪由表入里 ，侵犯肺中；或病理产物内生，停积肺中，无论是寒邪的凝滞，热邪的消灼，痰饮水湿的壅遏，均可使肺气闭阻，宣发、肃降失调，形成一派邪气亢盛，病情偏实的病机变化。由于肺实主要表现为宣降失调，故肺实的病机包括肺失宣发、肺失肃降、肺失宣降三个方面。

Chapter One

Impaired Diffusion of the Lung

The lung governs qì by upbearing and dissipating upward and outward. In this way, it perfuses its orifices, diffuses defense qì, promotes the uninhibited flow of the qì dynamic, disperses the fluids, warms and nourishes the skin and body hair, and secures and protects the fleshy exterior. When external evil invades, it usually assails the lung through the skin and body hair. For example, the "Treatise on Cough" in the *Sù Wèn* ("Plain Questions") explains: "The skin and body hair are connected to the lung. They are the first to contract evil qi, and the evil qì follows this connection." When disease evil invades the lung, it is most likely to impair diffusion. This manifests in impaired diffusion in the upper orifices, in impaired diffusion of lung-defense, or if it proceeds further, in such pathological changes as inhibited breathing.

肺失宣发

肺主气，向上向外升宣、发散以宣通肺窍，宣布卫气，流畅气机，布散津液，温煦滋养皮毛，固护肌表。外邪侵袭，多从皮毛而犯肺。如《素问•咳论》说："皮毛者，肺之合也。皮毛先受邪气，邪气从其合也。"病邪犯肺，最易导致肺失宣发，而呈现上窍失宣，肺卫失宣，进而引起呼吸不畅等病机变化。

1.1 Impaired Diffusion in the Upper Orifices

Both the nose and the throat serve as the upper orifices of the lung. As long as lung qì promotes diffusion and effusion, and distributes qì and liquid to the upper body, the upper orifices are free and disinhibited. However, when disease evil invades the lung, it impairs lung qì diffusion, resulting in blockage of the upper orifices, stoppage of lung qì, impaired distribution of the fluids, obstruction of the voice, and stasis bind in the upper orifices.

上窍失宣

鼻与喉均为肺之上窍。肺气宣发，气津上布，则上窍通利。病邪犯肺，宣发失职 ，使上窍失宣，可致肺气不通、津液不布、发音受阻、瘀结上窍。

1.1.1 Stoppage of Lung Qì

The chapter, "Vessel Measurement" in the *Líng Shū* ("The Magic Pivot") explains: "Lung qì penetrates to the nose. When the lung is harmonious, the nose is able to discern good and bad smells." This clearly indicates that a free flow of lung qì is the precondition for the nose's ability to perceive good and bad smells. When evil qì blocks the lung, it impairs diffusion and prevents lung qì from ascending and diffusing the nose. Qì stagnates inside the nose and contends with the fluids, thereby congesting the nostrils. This leads to nasal congestion, inability to differentiate between good and bad smells, and inhibited discharge of snivel.

The chapter, "Symptoms of Nasal Congestion" in the *Zhū Bìng Yuán Hòu Lùn* ("The Origin and Indicators of Disease") states:

> "The lung governs qì; its channel is the hand greater yīn vessel. Its qì penetrates to the nose. If the lung is harmonized, nose qì flows freely and the person can discern good and bad smells. But if wind or cold damage the internal organs and evil qì overwhelms the greater yīn channel, its qì smolders and accumulates in the nose. This results in fluid congestion and lack of regulated diffusion of qì in the nose. Therefore, such a person cannot discern good and bad smells, which means nasal congestion."

This illustrates specifically how wind-cold fettering the exterior prevents lung qì from diffusing and stops the flow of qì in the nose, which can lead to nasal congestion inhibiting the sense of smell.

The chapter, "Infantile Nasal Congestion" in the *Shèng Jì Zǒng Lù* ("Sages' Salvation Records") states: "Nasal congestion in small children means inhibition of lung qì." This indicates even more clearly that this disease is caused by the pathomechanism of lung qì stoppage. When lung qì fights with evil and surges upward with great effort, it can temporarily perfuse the blocked orifices. This results in sneezing. When lung qì fails to penetrate to the throat, qì and liquid congeal and stagnate, impeding the qì dynamic in the channels and network vessels. This can lead to sore throat.

This condition is treated by coursing wind and dissipating cold, and by diffusing the lung and disinhibiting the orifices. For mild patterns, *cōng chǐ tāng* (Scallion and Fermented Soybean Decoction) from the *Zhǒu Hòu Bèi Jí Fāng* ("Emergency Standby Remedies") is appropriate.

Cōng Chǐ Tāng 葱豉汤 (Scallion and Fermented Soybean Decoction)
cōng bái 葱白 (Allii Fistulosi Bulbus, scallion white) *dàn dòu chǐ* 淡豆豉 (Sojae Semen Praeparatum, fermented soybean)

For severe patterns, the best formula is *chuān xiōng chá tiáo sǎn* 川芎茶调散 (Tea Blended Chuanxiong Powder) from the *Zá Bìng Yuán Liú Xī Zhú* ("Incisive Light on the Source of Miscellaneous Disease"). This formula diffuses external evil, disinhibits lung qì, and frees the flow in the upper orifices. Thus the various symptoms of nasal congestion, inhibited discharge of snivel, and sneezing can be eliminated.

Chuān Xiōng Chá Tiáo Sǎn 川芎茶调散 (Tea-Blended Chuanxiong Powder)
chuān xiōng 川芎 (Chuanxiong Rhizoma, chuanxiong) *jīng jiè* 荆芥 (Schizonepetae Herba,) *fáng fēng* 防风 (Saposhnikoviae Radix,) *qiāng huó* 羌活 (Notopterygii Rhizoma et Radix, notopterygium) *bái zhǐ* 白芷 (Angelicae Dahuricae Radix, Dahurian angelica) *xì xīn* 细辛 (Asari Radix, asarum) *bò hé* 薄荷 (Menthae Herba,) *gān cǎo* 甘草 (Glycyrrhizae Radix, licorice)

The ingredients are pulverized and ingested mixed with tea.

肺气不通

《灵枢•脉度》说: "肺气通于鼻，肺和则鼻能知香臭矣。" 明确指出肺气通畅是鼻能闻香臭的前提。邪气闭肺，宣发失职，肺气不能上宣于鼻。气滞鼻中，与津液相搏，壅塞鼻道，可使鼻塞不通，香臭莫辨，涕出不畅。如《诸病源候论•鼻齆候》云: "肺主气，其经手太阴之脉也，其气通于鼻。若肺脏调和，则鼻气通利，而知香臭。若风冷伤于脏腑，而邪气乘于太阴之经，其气蕴积于鼻者，则津液壅塞，鼻气不宣调，故不知香臭，而为齆（鼻塞不通）也。" 直接阐明风寒外束，肺气不宣，鼻气不通，可致鼻塞不闻香臭。《圣济总录•小儿鼻齆塞》曰: "小儿鼻齆者，肺气不利也。" 更明确指出此病的病机是肺气不通。肺气与邪抗争，努力冲上，一时宣通闭塞之窍，则发为喷嚏。肺气不通于喉，气津凝滞，阻碍经络气机，可致喉痛。治宜疏风散寒，宣肺利窍。轻证宜《肘后方》葱豉汤（葱白、淡豆豉）；重证方选《杂病源流犀烛》川芎茶调散（川芎、荆芥、防风、羌活、白芷、细辛、薄荷、甘草为末，茶调下），外邪宣散，肺气通利，上窍得通，鼻塞、涕出不畅、喷嚏诸证可除。

1.1.2 Non-Distribution of Liquid and Qì

Among the humors, the lung is associated with snivel. When lung qì perfuses, the fluids are distributed upward. As a result, the nose orifice is moistened. But when external evil invades the lung and impairs the diffusion of lung qì, qì fails to distribute liquid to the nose and the nose is not moistened by the fluids. This can lead to dry nostrils. Wind-cold assailing the lung affects the transport of qì and liquid inside the nose. Qì and liquid stagnate and collect, amass and transform into snivel. When there is no heat boiling [the fluids], the result is runny nose with clear snivel.

The "Section on the Lung Viscus" in the *Shèng Jì Zǒng Lù* ("Sages' Salvation Records") explains:

> "It is said that a weakened lung viscus means damage by wind evil. Thus clear cold qì attacks the upper body, causing runny nose with clear snivel. The lung opens at the nose; among the humors, it is associated with snivel."

This quotation indicates how lung qì, when vacuous, easily contracts wind evil, which can lead to clear snivel. The chapter, "Profuse Snivel in Infants" in the same text further explains:

> "When lung qì is disharmonious, wind and cold can overwhelm it and cause obstruction and stoppage in the pathways of qì. As a result, wind and cold ascend with qì and cause blockage. Steaming, they turn into humor, and this humor in turn causes blockage in the lower body. The result is profuse snivel in the nose."

This explains in detail how impaired diffusion of the lung and obstruction of the qì pathways cause liquid to lodge in the nose, which results in the clear snivel.

This condition is treated by coursing wind and dissipating cold, and by eliminating dampness and checking snivel. The recommended formula is *xīn yí sǎn* (Magnolia Flower Powder) from the *Yán Shì Jì Shēng Fāng* ("Yan's Remedies for Curing All People") with additions.

Xīn Yí Sǎn 辛夷散 (Magnolia Flower Powder)
qiāng huó 羌活 (Notopterygii Rhizoma et Radix, notopterygium)
fáng fēng 防风 (Saposhnikoviae Radix, saposhnikovia)
gǎo běn 藁本 (Ligustici Rhizoma, Chinese lovage)
xì xīn 细辛(Asari Radix, asarum)
bái zhǐ 白芷 (Angelicae Dahuricae Radix, Dahurian angelica)
xīn yí 辛夷 (Magnoliae Flos, magnolia flower)
chuān xiōng 川芎 (Chuanxiong Rhizoma, chuanxiong)
shēng má 升麻 (Cimicifugae Rhizoma, cimicifuga)
mù tōng 木通 (Akebiae Trifoliatae Caulis, trifoliate akebia)
gān cǎo 甘草 (Glycyrrhizae Radix, licorice)

Plus:
tiān nán xīng 天南星 (Arisaematis Rhizoma, arisaema)
huā jiāo 花椒 (Zanthoxyli Pericarpium, zanthoxylum)

If disease is caused by a contraction of wind-heat evil and this boils, snivel transmutes and becomes thick and turbid. This results in runny nose with turbid snivel. If qì fails to distribute liquid to the throat, it causes reduced liquid and loss of moistening there. This results in dry throat. If fluids collect and are boiled by heat evil, phlegm and heat bind with each other and cause depression, steaming, and distress. This results in a sore red swollen throat. This condition is treated by coursing wind and diffusing the lung, and by clearing heat and disinhibiting the throat. The recommended formula is *xīn yí tāng* (Magnolia Flower Powder) from the *Yán Shì Jì Shēng Fāng* ("Yan's Remedies for Curing All People") with additions, which acts to eliminate turbid snivel and dry and sore throat.

Xīn Yí Tāng 辛夷汤 (Magnolia Flower Powder)

xīn yí 辛夷 (Magnoliae Flos, magnolia flower)
bò hé 薄荷 (Menthae Herba, mint)
chuān xiōng 川芎 (Chuanxiong Rhizoma, chuanxiong)
bái zhǐ 白芷 (Angelicae Dahuricae Radix, Dahurian angelica)
jú huā 菊花 (Chrysanthemi Flos, chrysanthemum)
qián hú 前胡 (Peucedani Radix, peucedanum)
shí gāo 石膏 (Gypsum Fibrosum, gypsum)
shēng dì huáng 生地黄 (Rehmanniae Radix, rehmannia)
bái zhú 白朮 (Atractylodis Macrocephalae Rhizoma, white atractylodes)
chì fú ling 赤茯苓 (Poria Rubra, red poria)
chén pí 陈皮 (Citri Reticulatae Pericarpium, tangerine peel)
gān cǎo 甘草 (Glycyrrhizae Radix, licorice)
Plus:
jié gěng 桔梗 (Platycodonis Radix, platycodon)
niú bàng zǐ 牛蒡子 (Arctii Fructus, arctium)

津气不布

肺在液为涕，肺气宣通，津液上布，则鼻窍润泽。外邪犯肺，肺气失宣，气不布津于鼻，鼻失津液滋润，可致鼻孔干燥。若风寒袭肺，影响鼻中气津输布，气滞津停，蓄积化涕，又无热煎熬，则鼻流清涕。《圣济总录•肺脏门》说：“论曰肺藏虚弱，为风邪所伤，则清冷之气上攻，而鼻流清涕。盖肺开窍于鼻，在液为涕也。”指出肺气虚弱，易感风邪，可致清涕。《圣济总录•小儿多涕》又说："肺气不和，风冷乘之，使气道遏而不通，则风冷与气上畀（音闭），蒸而为液，其液复畀于下，故令鼻多涕。"则详细阐述肺失宣发，阻遏气道，津停鼻中而引起清涕的病机变化。治宜疏风散寒，除湿止涕。方选《济生方》辛夷散（羌活、防风、藁本、细辛、白芷、辛夷、升麻、木通、甘草）加南星、川椒。

若受风热之邪煎熬，涕变稠浊，则流浊涕。若气不布津于喉，津少失濡，则喉中干燥。若津液停聚，热邪煎熬，痰热互结，郁蒸逼迫，则为咽喉红肿疼痛。治宜疏风宣肺，清热利咽。方选《济生方》辛夷汤（辛夷、薄荷、川芎、白芷、菊花、前胡、石膏、生地、白术、赤茯苓、陈皮、甘草）加桔梗、牛蒡子，浊涕、喉干、咽痛可除。

1.1.3 Obstruction of the Voice

When lung qì flows freely in the throat, the voice is able to resonate. When evil qì invades the lung, it impairs diffusion of the upper orifices. Lung qì is unable to agitate the throat and epiglottis. This can lead to muteness and loss of voice.

The "Treatise on Speechlessness with Anxiety and Rage" in the *Líng Shū* ("The Magic Pivot") explains: "When a person is suddenly speechless, cold qì has lodged in the epiglottis." The "Schema of Miscellaneous Patterns; Loss of Voice" in the *Jǐng Yuè Quán Shū* (Jǐng-Yuè's Complete Compendium") states: "It is owing to qì that sound is emitted. When the lung is diseased, qì is despoliated. For this reason, qì is the door to the voice." Both these sources shed light on the pathomechanism by which an obstruction by external evil impairs the diffusion of lung qì and prevents qì from surging upward, which affects the voice.

This condition is treated by diffusing the lung and disinhibiting qì. Based on differences in the nature of the external evil, different exterior-resolving formulas are selected. In cases of wind-cold fettering the exterior, the appropriate formula is *sān ào tāng* (Rough and Ready Three Decoction) from the *Tài Píng Huì Mín Hé Jì Jú Fāng* (Tài-Píng Imperial Grace Pharmacy Formulas) with additions.

Sān Ào Tāng 三拗汤 (Rough and Ready Three Decoction)
má huáng 麻黄 (Ephedrae Herba, ephedra) *xìng rén* 杏仁 (Armeniacae Semen, apricot kernel) *gān cǎo* 甘草 (Glycyrrhizae Radix, licorice)

Plus:
jié gěng 桔梗 (Platycodonis Radix, platycodon)
mù hú dié 木蝴蝶 (Oroxyli Semen, oroxylum)

For externally contracted wind-heat, the recommended formula is *qīng yàn níng fèi tāng* (Clear the Throat and Calm the Lung Decoction) from the textbook *Fāng Jì Xué* ("Formulas") with additions.

Qīng Yàn Níng Fèi Tāng 清咽宁肺汤 (Clear the Throat and Calm the Lung Decoction)
jié gěng 桔梗 (Platycodonis Radix, platycodon)
qián hú 前胡 (Peucedani Radix, peucedanum)
sāng bái pí 桑白皮 (Mori Cortex, mulberry root bark)
huáng qín 黄芩 (Scutellariae Radix, scutellaria)
zhī zǐ 栀子 (Gardeniae Fructus, gardenia)
zhī mǔ 知母 (Anemarrhenae Rhizoma, anemarrhena)
bèi mǔ 贝母 (Fritillariae Bulbus, fritillaria)
gān cǎo 甘草 (Glycyrrhizae Radix, licorice)
Plus:
pàng dà hǎi 胖大海 (Sterculiae Lychnophorae Semen, sterculia)
chán tuì 蝉蜕 (Cicadae Periostracum, cicada molting)
niú bàng zǐ 牛蒡子 (Arctii Fructus, arctium)
pí pá yè 枇杷叶 (Eriobotryae Folium, loquat)

发音受阻

肺气通于喉，则声音得彰。邪气犯肺，上窍失宣，肺气不能鼓动喉头会厌，可致声哑、失音。《灵枢•忧恚无言论》说："人卒然无言者，寒气客于会厌。"《景岳全书•杂证谟•声瘖》："声由气而发，肺病则气夺，此气为声音之户也。"均阐明外邪闭阻，肺气失宣，气不上冲而影响发声的病机。治宜宣肺利气，并根据外邪的性质不同，选用不同解表方剂。如风寒束表用《和剂局方》三拗汤（麻黄、杏仁、甘草）加桔梗、蝉衣、木蝴蝶；外感风热用《方剂学》清咽宁肺汤（桔梗、前胡、桑白皮、黄芩、山栀、知母、贝母、甘草）加胖大海、蝉衣、牛蒡子、枇杷叶。

1.1.4 Stasis Bind in the Upper Orifices

When the body contracts evil qì of the six excesses, lung qì loses its ability to diffuse, and qì then fails to promote the flow of blood. Alternatively, an internal exuberance of visceral yáng qì can engender phlegm-fire, which rises and congests the throat, prevents qì from moving blood, and causes qì stagnation and blood stasis in the upper orifices. If qì and blood stagnate in the throat, the result is sore swollen throat, inhibited swallowing in the throat, and choking when drinking water. When qì and blood stagnate in the epiglottis, the epiglottal blood network vessels fill up, and it fails to close completely. This results in nodes in the epiglottis, hoarse voice, and perhaps the sensation of foreign matter.

Qì and blood stasis obstruction manifests in a dark purple tongue with stasis macules or stasis speckles, and a rough pulse. The chapter, "The Throat" in the *Yī Biǎn* ("Lancing Stones of Medicine") states:

> "The throat is the passageway for food and drink, and for breathing. It is situated on top of the internal organs. Regardless of which channel is affected by evil, it can always implicate the upper body… All diseases of the throat are associated with fire. There are those where upper burner fire exuberates, and there are those where lower burner fire surges. They all lead to phlegm-drool and qì-blood gathering and binding, which causes swelling, pain, and block."

An external invasion of evil qì of the six excesses engenders internal phlegm-fire, which flames upward. This can equally impede the movement of qì and blood in the throat and cause qì stagnation and blood stasis. Consequently, they stagnate and bind in the upper orifices, causing a sore swollen uncomfortable throat.

This condition is treated by moving qì and quickening blood, and by resolving toxin and disinhibiting the throat. The recommended formula is *huì yàn zhú yū tāng* (Epiglottis Stasis-Expelling Decoction) from the *Yī Lín Gǎi Cuò* ("Correction of Errors in Medical Classics") with additions.

Huì Yàn Zhú Yū Tāng 会厌逐瘀汤 (Epiglottis Stasis-Expelling Decoction)

táo rén 桃仁 (Persicae Semen, peach kernel)
hóng huā 红花 (Carthami Flos, carthamus)
shēng dì huáng 生地黄 (Rehmanniae Radix, rehmannia)
dāng guī 当归 (Angelicae Sinensis Radix, Chinese angelica)
chì sháo 赤芍 (Paeoniae Radix Rubra)
chái hú 柴胡 (Bupleuri Radix, bupleurum)
xuán shēn 玄参 (Scrophulariae Radix, scrophularia)
zhǐ qiào (*ké*) 枳壳 (Aurantii Fructus, bitter orange)
jié gěng 桔梗 (Platycodonis Radix, platycodon)
gān cǎo 甘草 (Glycyrrhizae Radix, licorice)

Plus:
jīn yín huā 金银花 (Lonicerae Flos, lonicera)
sāng yè 桑叶 (Mori Folium, mulberry leaf)
lián qiào 连翘 (Forsythiae Fructus, forsythia)
chán tuì 蝉蜕 (Cicadae Periostracum, cicada molting)

瘀结上窍

外感六淫邪气，肺气失宣，气不推动血行，或内脏阳气亢盛，化生痰火，上壅咽喉，使气不行血，气血瘀滞于上窍。若气血瘀滞于咽喉，则引起咽喉肿痛、吞咽不利、饮水则呛；气血瘀滞于会厌，会厌血络充盈，关闭不全，则会厌结节、声音嘶哑、或有异物感；气血瘀阻，则舌质紫暗、有瘀斑瘀点、脉涩。如《医碥•咽喉》曰："咽喉为饮食、呼吸之通路，居脏腑之上，不论何经之邪，皆得上干。…咽喉之病皆属于火，有上焦火盛者，有下焦火冲者，以致痰涎气血聚结，肿痛闭塞。"六淫邪气外侵，内生痰火上炎，均会咽喉阻碍气血运行，气滞血瘀，瘀结上窍，则会引起咽喉肿痛不适。治宜行气活血，解毒利咽。方选《医林改错》会厌逐瘀汤。药用（桃仁、红花、生地、当归、赤芍、柴胡、玄参，枳壳、桔梗、甘草）加银花、桑叶、连翘、蝉衣。

Literature Review of Impaired Diffusion in the Upper Orifices

📖 *Sì Shèng Xīn Yuán* ("The Four Sages' Original Heart"), "The Source of Nose Disease"

> "Nose disease means that the hand greater yīn is not cleared. The lung opens at the nose. It is in charge of defense qì and of downbearing and constraint. It houses ancestral qì in the chest, is the root of defensive yáng, links up with the heart channel, and moves the breath, which exits and enters through the nose. When the lung performs downbearing, ancestral qì is depurated and the nose cleared. When lung qì counterflows, ancestral qì is obstructed and the nose congested."

This quotation describes how the pathomechanism of nasal congestion is caused by counterflow ascent of lung qì and obstruction of ancestral qì. In actuality, counterflow ascent of lung qì is mostly caused by an invasion of external evil, lung qì depression block, and impaired lung diffusion.

📖 *Zhū Bìng Yuán Hòu Lùn* ("The Origin and Indicators of Disease"), "Symptoms of Snivel in the Nose"

> "When liquid, humor, snivel, and spittle contract heat, they become dry; when they contract cold, they flow and spill uncontrollably. Lung qì

flows to the nose. When its viscus is cold, the cold follows qì up into the nose. Therefore, the fluids cannot be contained."

This quotation explains that when cold evil invades the lung and the lung fails to diffuse, fluids collect in the nose and spill out of it, which creates clear snivel.

🕮 *Qiān Jīn Yào Fāng* ("A Thousand Gold Pieces Prescriptions"), "Wind Choke"

"When the qì of wind-cold settles in the center and stagnates instead of effusing, it causes loss of voice and inability to speak. It is all due to wind evil."

This quotation points out that externally contract wind-cold can prevent lung qì from diffusing and thereby lead to loss of voice.

🕮 *Gǔ Jīn Yī Tǒng Dà Quán* ("The Complete Compendium of Medical Works, Ancient and Modern"), "The Voice"

"The lung belongs to metal. It governs depuration and on the outside is in charge of the cutaneous interstices. As a result of an external contraction of wind-cold, heat is depressed inside the body. This prevents lung-metal from clearing and manifests in cough and muteness."

This quotation describes how external cold and internal heat cause lung qì depression block, impaired depuration, and loss of lung qì diffusion, which can lead to loss of voice.

🕮 *Hǒu Kē Jí Yè* ("Throat Department: Collection to Keep Under Your Arm"), "Throat Impediment"

"The larynx governs heavenly qì and belongs to lung-metal. Change makes it dry; when it is dry, it becomes rough and therefore blocked. The pharynx governs earthly qì and belongs to spleen-earth. Change makes it damp; when it is damp, it becomes swollen and distended. Whenever fire is depressed in the upper burner, it leads to phlegm-drool and qì-blood binding and gathering, to swelling and outthrusting in the larynx and pharynx, and hence to numbness, itching, and pain."

This quotation describes the pathomechanism by which numerous causes impede the movement of qì and blood and congeal static blood in the throat, resulting in swelling, distention, and pain.

文献评述

《四圣心源•鼻病根源》曰："鼻病者，手太阴之不清也。肺开窍于鼻，司卫气而降敛，宗气在胸，卫阳为本，贯心脉而行呼吸，出入鼻窍者也，肺降则宗气清肃而鼻通，肺气逆则宗气壅阻而鼻塞。"阐述鼻塞的病机为肺气上逆，宗气壅阻。实际上多因外邪侵袭，肺气闭郁，肺失宣发而使肺气上逆。

《诸病源候论•鼻涕候》曰："夫津液涕唾，得热则干燥，得冷则流溢不能收。肺气通于鼻，其脏有冷，冷随气入乘于鼻，故使津液不能收。"说明寒冷之邪犯肺，肺失宣发，津液停留鼻中，流溢鼻外，而成清涕。

《千金要方•风懿》曰："风寒之气客于中，滞而不能发，故瘖不能言及瘖症失声，皆风邪所为。"指出外感风寒，肺气失宣，可致失音。

《古今医统大全•声音》曰："肺者属金，主清肃，外司皮腠。风寒外感者，热郁于内，则肺金不清，咳嗽而哑。"论述外寒内热，肺气闭郁，清肃失职，肺气失宣，可致失音。

《喉科集腋•喉痹》曰："喉主天气，属肺金，变动为燥，燥则涩而闭；咽主地气，属脾土，变动为湿，湿则肿而胀；皆火郁上焦，致痰涎气血结聚，咽喉肿达于外，麻木痒痛。"论述多种原因阻碍气血运行，瘀血凝滞咽喉而引起肿胀疼痛的病机。

Summary of Impaired Diffusion in the Upper Orifices

1. Stoppage of Lung Qì

   Congestion in the nostrils: Nasal congestion and stoppage, inability to differentiate between good and bad smells, inhibited discharge of snivel.

   Lung qì fighting evil: Sneezing.

   Qì and liquid obstructing the throat: Sore throat.

2. Non-Distribution of Liquid and Qì

   Loss of moistening: Dry nose, itchy throat.

   Wind-cold assailing the lung, qì stagnation and liquid collection: Runny nose with clear snivel.

   Wind-heat invading the lung, evil boiling the fluids: Runny nose with turbid snivel.

   Phlegm and heat binding with each other; lying depressed, steaming and distressing the throat: Sore red swollen throat.

3. Obstruction of the Voice

   Muteness, loss of voice.

4. Stasis Bind in the Upper Orifices

   Stagnation in the throat: Sore swollen throat, disinhibited swallowing, choking when drinking water.

   Stagnation in the epiglottis: Epiglottal nodes, hoarse voice, perhaps with sensation of foreign matter.

上窍失宣
肺气不通——
壅塞鼻道—鼻塞不通、香臭不辨、涕出不畅。
肺气抗邪—喷嚏。
气津阻咽—咽喉疼痛。
津气不布——
失于滋润—鼻干、喉痒。
风寒袭肺，气滞津停—鼻流清涕。
风热犯肺，邪煎津液—鼻流浊涕。
痰热互结，郁蒸逼迫—咽喉红肿疼痛。
法音受阻——声哑、失音。
瘀结上窍——
瘀滞咽喉—咽喉肿痛、吞咽不利、饮水则呛。
瘀滞会厌—会厌结节、声音嘶哑、或有异物感。

1.2 Impaired Diffusion of Lung-Defense

The lung governs diffusion and spreads defense qì and the fluids out over the surface of the body. By "warming the divided flesh, filling the skin, and fattening the interstices," it combats external evil. When evil from the six excesses invades the human body through the mouth, nose, skin, and body hair, it congeals and blocks lung-defense. This obstructs the diffusing mechanism of lung qì and impairs the function of regulating the defensive exterior, resulting in the pathomechanism of impaired diffusion of lung-defense.

Based on differences in the nature of the disease evil and individual factors, the development of this pathomechanism can follow particular tendencies after the loss of lung-defense diffusion. Most important among these are: Depression of defense qì; disharmony in the interstices; inhibited flow of channel qì; loss of moistening due to scant liquid; and water qì flooding and spilling.

肺卫失宣

肺主宣发，将卫气和津液布敷体表以“温分肉，充皮肤，肥腠理”，抗御外邪。六淫之邪由口鼻皮毛侵犯人体，凝闭肺卫，肺气宣发之机受阻，卫表调节功能失职，则引起肺卫失宣的病机。由于病邪性质和个体因素的差异，肺卫失宣后其病机发展趋势各有侧重，主要有卫气遏郁、腠理失调、经气不利、津少失濡、水气泛溢等几个方面。

1.2.1 Depression of Defense Qì

When the evil qì of any of the six excesses (wind, cold, summerheat, dampness, dryness, fire) invades the fleshy exterior, it can cause depression of defense qì. The reason for this is that an assault by the six excesses on the exterior arouses defense qì to fight against evil. As it single-handedly dispels evil out of the body, however, it can also be worn out and entrapped by evil qì. If this happens, defense yáng loses its ability to warm the fleshy exterior. This results in aversion to cold. When defense yáng fights evil, yáng floats to the fleshy exterior. Since it cannot be discharged to the outside, it is depressed in the body's exterior. Consequently, superabundant qì causes heat effusion. When evil qì damages the body's defense and struggles simultaneously with defense and with yáng, aversion to cold and heat effusion mnaifest simultaneously. When cold evil in this process assails the exterior, its contracting and congealing nature not only directly depresses defense qì, but at the same time it can contract the body hair and sweat pores, block the interstices, and impede the movement of defense qì. For this reason, cold evil is the key pathomechanism that leads to depression of defense qì, with the symptoms of aversion to cold and heat effusion being particularly obvious.

This condition is treated by dispelling and dissipating wind-cold, and by effusing straying defense qì. The recommended formula is *sū qiāng yǐn* (Notopterygii and Perilla Beverage) from the *Sōng Fēng Shuō Yì* ("Song-Feng's Discussion on Epidemics").

Sū Qiāng Yǐn 苏羌饮 (Notopterygii and Perilla Beverage)
zǐ sū yè 紫苏叶 (Perillae Folium, perilla leaf) *qiāng huó* 羌活 (Notopterygii Rhizoma et Radix, notopterygium) *fáng fēng* 防风 (Saposhnikoviae Radix, saposhnikovia) *chén pí* 陈皮 (Citri Reticulatae Pericarpium, tangerine peel) *shēng jiāng* 生姜 (Zingiberis Rhizoma Recens, fresh ginger) *cōng bái* 葱白 (Allii Fistulosi Bulbus, scallion white) *dàn dòu chǐ* 淡豆豉 (Sojae Semen Praeparatum, fermented soybean)

卫气遏郁

风寒暑湿燥火等六淫邪气侵犯肌表，均可引起卫气遏郁。这是因为，六淫袭表，卫气奋起抗邪，在祛邪外出的同时，自身亦受到邪气的困顿，反被邪气所遏。卫气被遏，卫阳失却对肌表的温煦则恶寒；卫阳抗邪，阳浮肌表，不得外泄，郁于体表，气有余而发热；邪气伤卫，与卫阳抗争同时进行，则恶寒与发热同时并见。其中寒邪袭表，其收引、凝滞之性不仅可直接遏郁卫气，还可通过收缩皮毛、汗孔，闭塞腠理而阻碍卫气运行，故寒邪是引起卫气遏郁的主要病机，恶寒发热之症尤为显著。治宜祛散风寒，发越卫气。方选《松峰说疫》苏羌饮（紫苏、羌活、防风、陈皮、生姜、葱白、淡豆豉）。

1.2.2 Disharmony in the Interstices

The interstices are the grain in the skin, flesh, and bowels and viscera. They are the gates through which bodily humor percolates and qì and blood flow, and they are regulated by the lung's defense qì. When evil qì invades the lung, lung defense is unable to diffuse. This can easily lead to irregular opening and closing of the interstices.

Cold evil tends to cause blocks in the interstices. Cold is a yīn evil and governs contracture and tautness, congealing and stagnation. It can cause the skin and body hair to contract and retract and the sweat pores to close. When the interstices close and fail to open, lung defense qì is unable to effuse the fluids and discharge them outwards. This can lead to absence of sweating and aversion to cold.

The "Treatise on Pain" in the *Sù Wèn* ("Plain Questions") explains: "Cold results in blocked interstices and in qì failing to move." This expresses precisely the pathomechanism by which cold qì blocks defense qì and impairs diffusion in the interstices.

This condition is treated by acrid warming and by promoting sweating. The recommended formula is *má huáng tāng* (Ephedra Decoction) from the *Shāng Hán Lùn* ("On Cold Damage").

Má Huáng Tāng 麻黄汤 (Ephedra Decoction)
má huáng 麻黄 (Ephedrae Herba, ephedra)
guì zhī 桂枝 (Cinnamomi Ramulus, cinnamon twig)
xìng rén 杏仁 (Armeniacae Semen, apricot kernel)
gān cǎo 甘草 (Glycyrrhizae Radix, licorice)

The evils of wind, summerheat, or heat can cause the interstices to open and discharge. Wind is a yáng evil, and its nature is to open and discharge. When it invades from the outside, it can easily damage defense qì. As a result, defense yáng is unable to fill the skin and fatten the interstices. Opening and closing break down and the mysterious mansions (i.e. sweat pores) lose their tightness. Consequently, we observe sweating with aversion to wind.

The chapter, "Straight Treatment of Wind Strike" in the *Shāng Hán Sù Yuán Jì* ("Traced Collections on Cold Damage") explains this directly: "Wind strike means that wind damages defense. When wind evil invades through the body hair pores, defense qì is unable to manage their opening and closure with constancy and the mysterious mansions fail to close. Hence sweating ensues."

This condition is treated by coursing and dissipating wind evil, and by harmonizing construction and defense. The recommended formula is *guì zhī tāng* (Cinnamon Twig Decoction) from the *Shāng Hán Lùn* ("On Cold Damage").

Guì Zhī Tāng 桂枝汤 (Cinnamon Twig Decoction)
guì zhī 桂枝 (Cinnamomi Ramulus, cinnamon twig) *sháo yào* 芍药 (Paeoniae Radix, peony) *shēng jiāng* 生姜 (Zingiberis Rhizoma Recens) *dà zǎo* 大枣 (Jujubae Fructus, jujube) *zhì gān cǎo* 炙甘草 (Glycyrrhizae Radix Praeparata, mix-fried licorice)

Summerheat and heat are also yáng evils. When they invade the lung, intense internal heat lies depressed, steaming upward and outward. It can loosen the interstices, which causes outward discharge of the fluids and incessant sweating.

This is precisely the meaning of the following sentence in the "Treatise on Pain" in the *Sù Wèn* ("Plain Questions"): "Intense heat results in opening of the interstices, free flow of construction and defense, great discharge of sweat, and therefore discharge of qì."

This condition is treated by clearing heat and resolving summerheat, and by harmonizing the interstices. The recommended method is *qīng liáng dí shǔ fǎ* (Cool Clearing Summerheat-Flushing Method) from the *Shí Bìng Lùn* ("On Seasonal Diseases").

Qīng Liáng Dí Shǔ Fǎ 清凉涤暑法 (Cool Clearing Summerheat-Flushing Method)
bái biǎn dòu 白扁豆 (Lablab Semen Album, lablab) *qīng hāo* 青蒿 (Artemisiae Annuae Herba, sweet wormwood) *lián qiào* 连翘 (Forsythiae Fructus, forsythia) *fú líng* 茯苓 (Poria, poria) *huá shí* 滑石 (Talcum, talcum) *tōng cǎo* 通草 (Tetrapanacis Medulla, rice-paper plant pith) *gān cǎo* 甘草 (Glycyrrhizae Radix, licorice)

From this we can see that wind evil opening and discharging, and summerheat or heat upbearing and dissipating involve different pathomechanisms, but can both affect the opening and closing of the mysterious mansions and the functioning of the interstices.

腠理失调

腠理是皮肤、肌肉、脏腑之纹理，是渗泄体液，流通气血的门户，受肺卫之气的调节。邪气犯肺，肺卫失宣，易引起腠理开阖失调。

寒邪易使腠理闭塞。寒为阴邪而主收引、凝滞，能使皮毛收缩，汗孔关闭，腠理阖而不开，肺卫之气不能宣发津液外泄，可致无汗、恶寒之症。《素问•举痛论》说："寒则腠理闭，气不行。"正好清楚地揭示了寒气闭塞卫气，腠理失宣的病机。治宜辛温发汗。方选《伤寒论》麻黄汤（麻黄、桂枝、杏仁、甘草）。

风、暑、热邪可致腠理开泄。风为阳邪，其性开泄，由外侵袭，易伤卫气。卫阳不能充皮肤，肥腠理，开阖失司，玄府失密，故见汗出恶风之症。正如《伤寒溯源集•中风正治》所说："中风，风伤卫也。风邪袭于毛孔，卫气不能司其开阖之常，玄府不闭，故汗出。"治宜疏散风邪，调和营卫。方选《伤寒论》桂枝汤（桂枝、芍药、生姜、大枣、炙甘草）。暑、热亦为阳邪，暑热犯肺，里热炽盛，郁蒸升散，可使腠理疏松，津液外泄，汗出不止。即《素问•举痛论》"炅则腠理开，营卫通，汗大泄，故气泄"之意。治宜清热解暑，调和腠理。方选《时病论》清凉涤暑法（白扁豆、青蒿、连翘、茯苓、滑石、通草、甘草）。由此可见，风邪开泄，暑、热升散，虽然病机有别，但均能使玄府失其开阖，而致肌腠失调。

1.2.3. Inhibited Flow of Channel Qì

When the six excesses assail the exterior and prevent lung defense from diffusing, the exterior defense becomes insecure, and the channels and network vessels empty. Evil qì exploits the vacuity and enters, impeding the movement of channel qì. This leads to inhibited flow of channel qì, which manifests in pain as the main symptom.

Wind-evil is swift and changeable. When it invades from the outside, it obstructs the channels and network vessels and blocks channel qì. The obstruction is of unfixed location, frequently shifting and never residing in one place for long. Therefore, the result is wandering pain in the head, whole body, joints, and flesh. At the same time, the inhibited flow of channel qì causes a loss of nourishment in the channels and vessels, which leads to hypertonicity and engenders wind. This manifests in deviated eyes and mouth, numbness of the skin, rigidity of the limbs, spasms in the hands and feet, and similar symptoms of stirring wind.

The chapter, "Pulse Symptoms and Treatments of Wind Strike Joint Running Disease" in the *Jīn Guì Yào Lüè* ("Essential Prescriptions of the Golden Coffer") states:

> "When wind causes disease such as hemiplegia or paralysis of the arms only, this means impediment. The pulse will be faint and rapid. Wind strike makes this happen… Floating [is related to] blood vacuity, to emptiness in the network vessels, and to bandit evil failing to drain. Whether on the left or on the right, when evil qì slackens, right qì immediately tenses. Right qì makes the evil taut, which causes deviation and paralysis of the face."

This describes the pathomechanism by which wind evil invading the channels and network vessels leads to inhibited flow of channel qì, hypertonicity in the channels, and stirring wind.

This condition is treated by dispelling wind and eliminating dampness, and by quickening blood and freeing the network vessels. The recommended formula is *dà qín jiāo tāng* (Large Gentian Decoction) from the *Bǎo Mìng Jí* ("Collection on Preserving Life").

Dà Qín Jiāo Tāng 大秦艽汤 (Large Gentian Decoction)
qín jiāo 秦艽 (Gentianae Macrophyllae Radix, large gentian)
fáng fēng 防风 (Saposhnikoviae Radix, saposhnikovia)
qiāng huó 羌活 (Notopterygii Rhizoma et Radix, notopterygium)
dú huó 独活 (Angelicae Pubescentis Radix, pubescent angelica)
bái zhǐ 白芷 (Angelicae Dahuricae Radix, Dahurian angelica)
xì xīn 细辛 (Asari Radix, asarum)
chuān xiōng 川芎 (Chuanxiong Rhizoma, chuanxiong)
dāng guī 当归 (Angelicae Sinensis Radix, Chinese angelica)
bái sháo 白芍 (Paeoniae Radix Alba, white peony)
shēng dì huáng 生地黄 (Rehmanniae Radix, rehmannia)
shú dì huáng 熟地黄 (Rehmanniae Radix Praeparata, cooked rehmannia)
bái zhú 白术 (Atractylodis Macrocephalae Rhizoma, white atractylodes)
fú líng 茯苓 (Poria, poria)
huáng qín 黄芩 (Scutellariae Radix, scutellaria)
shí gāo 石膏 (Gypsum Fibrosum, gypsum)
gān cǎo 甘草 (Glycyrrhizae Radix, licorice)

Cold is a yīn evil and governs contracture and tautness, congealing and stagnating. When cold evil assails the channels and network vessels, channel qì congeals and stagnates, and the channel vessels contract and tighten. This leads to severe pain, manifesting in symptoms like headache and painful stiff nape, generalized aching and lumbar pain, joint pain throughout the body, and hypertonicity of the extremities.

This is explained directly in the "Treatise on Pain" in the *Sù Wèn* ("Plain Questions"):

> "As cold qì enters the channels, it gradually slows down the flow of qì and blood therein to the point of dribbling and eventually not moving at all. If it settles outside the vessels, the result is scantiness of blood; if it settles inside the vessels, the result is stoppage of qì. For this reason, pain suddenly occurs."

Stoppage resulting in pain is the key pathomechanism of cold evil stagnating and congesting channel qì. The chapter, "Harmonizing and Resolving" in the *Shì Yī Dé Xiào Fāng* ("Effective Formula From a Family Tradition"), "Adult Medicine and Miscellaneous Diseases" also explains:

> "When entering the interstices, [cold evil] causes the person to suffer from a heavy body, aching pain in the limb joints, and hypertonicity of the nape and neck…Whenever a person experiences these signs, failure to move, resolve, and disinhibit [the evil] will remain latent in the channels and network vessels and change continuously."

This quotation explains the pathomechanism by which cold evil invading the interstices and entering deeply into the channels and network vessels can impede channel qì, which results in headache, body pain, and hypertonicity of the nape and neck.

This condition is treated by dispelling wind and dissipating cold, and by warming yáng and freeing the network vessels. The recommended formula is *xiǎo xù mìng tāng* (Minor Life-Prolonging Decoction) from the *Qiān Jīn Yào Fāng* ("A Thousand Gold Pieces Prescriptions").

Xiǎo Xù Mìng Tāng 小续命汤 (Minor Life-Prolonging Decoction)
má huáng 麻黄 (Ephedrae Herba, ephedra) *guì zhī* 桂枝 (Cinnamomi Ramulus, cinnamon twig) *xìng rén* 杏仁 (Armeniacae Semen, apricot kernel) *bái sháo* 白芍 (Paeoniae Radix Alba, white peony) *shēng jiāng* 生姜 (Zingiberis Rhizoma Recens, fresh ginger) *fáng fēng* 防风 (Saposhnikoviae Radix, saposhnikovia) *fáng jǐ* 防已 (Stephaniae Tetrandrae Radix, fangji) *chuān xiōng* 川芎 (Chuanxiong Rhizoma, chuanxiong) *rén shēn* 人参 (Ginseng Radix, ginseng) *fù zǐ* 附子 (Aconiti Radix Lateralis Praeparata, aconite) *gān cǎo* 甘草 (Glycyrrhizae Radix, licorice)

Dampness by its nature belongs to yīn. When it assails the channels and network vessels, it is most likely to impede the qì dynamic. Moreover, as its nature is sticky, stagnating, heavy, and fixed, it usually causes channel qì to adhere. Thus it becomes entangled and difficult to resolve. Because the resulting pain has the distinctive trait of being heavy, fixed, and aching, you may observe the various symptoms of head heavy as if swathed, generalized heaviness, encumbrance, and fatigue, and heavy and fixed aching pain in the limbs and body, flesh, and joints.

The chapter, "Discussing the Treatment of Dampness Patterns" in the *Lèi Zhèng Zhì Cái* ("Systematized Patterns with Clear-Cut Treatments") states:

> "Whenever it is located in the fleshy exterior, the result is aversion to cold and spontaneous sweating. When it is located in the divided flesh, the result is numbness and puffy swelling, heaviness like a mountain, inability to freely turn sides, swelling of the lumbus and knees, joint and bone pain, inhibited urination, and sloppy stools."

The section, "The Three Qì of Heat, Dampness, and Summer-Heat" in the ("Axioms of Medicine") also explains:

> "When yáng is exuberant in the human body, it feels light and graceful. But when dampness exuberates, the body is affected by feeling heavy like a mountain, with pain in the hundred vessels and inability to turn sides."

Both these sources discuss the pathomechanism by which dampness evil stagnating channel qì results in soreness and heavy pain in the body.

This condition is treated by dispelling wind and dissipating cold, and by eliminating dampness and freeing the network vessels. The recommended formula is *qiāng huó shèng shī tāng* (Notopterygium Dampness-Overcoming Decoction) from the *Nèi Wài Shāng Biàn Huò Lùn* ("Clarification of Perpexities About Internal and External Damage").

Qiāng Huó Shèng Shī Tāng 羌活胜湿汤 (Notopterygium Dampness-Overcoming Decoction)
qiāng huó 羌活 (Notopterygii Rhizoma et Radix, notopterygium) *dú huó* 独活 (Angelicae Pubescentis Radix, pubescent angelica) *fáng fēng* 防风 (Saposhnikoviae Radix, saposhnikovia) *gǎo běn* 藁本 (Ligustici Rhizoma, Chinese lovage) *chuān xiōng* 川芎 (Chuanxiong Rhizoma, chuanxiong) *màn jīng zǐ* 蔓荆子 (Viticis Fructus, vitex) *gān cǎo* 甘草 (Glycyrrhizae Radix, licorice)

经气不利

六淫袭表，肺卫失宣，卫表不固，经络空虚，邪气乘虚而入，阻碍经气运行，导致经气不利，表现以疼痛为主的症状。

风邪善行而数变，风邪外袭，阻滞经络，闭塞经气，阻闭的部位游移不定，善动不居，故引起头身、关节、肌肉游走性疼痛。并因经气不利，经脉失养，诱发经脉挛急而生风，则出现口眼歪斜、肌肤麻木、肢体强直、手足痉挛等动风的症状。如《金匮要略•中风历节病脉证并治》曰："夫风之为病，当半身不遂，或但臂不遂者，此为痹，脉微而数，中风使然。"同时又说："浮者血虚，络脉空虚，贼邪不泻，或左或右，邪气反缓，正气即急，正气引邪，㖞僻不遂。"阐述了风邪侵犯经络，经气不利，经脉挛急而引起动风的病机。治宜祛风除湿，活血通络。方选《保命集》大秦艽汤（秦艽、防风、羌活、独活、白芷、细辛、川芎、当归、白芍、生地黄、熟地黄、白术、茯苓、黄芩、石膏、甘草）。

寒为阴邪，主收引、凝滞。寒邪侵袭经络，经气凝滞，经脉收引，引起剧烈疼痛，表现为头项强痛、身疼腰痛、周身骨节疼痛，手足拘急等症。正如《素问•举痛论》所说："寒气入经而稽迟，泣而不行。客于脉外则血少，客于脉中则气不通，故卒然而痛。"不通而痛，是寒邪滞塞经气的主要病机。《世医得效方•大方脉杂医科•和解》又说：寒邪"入于腠理，使人身体沉重，肢节酸疼，项背拘急，…凡此之证，若不便行解利，伏留经络，传变不已。"说明寒邪侵入腠理，深入经络，可阻碍经气，引起头身疼痛，项背拘急的病机。治宜祛风散寒，温阳通络。方选《千金要方》小续命汤（麻黄、桂枝、杏仁、白芍、生姜、防风、防己、川芎、人参、附子、甘草）。

湿性属阴，侵袭经络，最易阻碍气机。又因其性粘滞，重着，常使经气胶着，缠绵难解。所致疼痛以重着、酸痛为特征，可见头重如裹、身重困倦、肢体肌肉关节酸痛、重着不移诸症。如《类证治裁•湿证论治》曰："或在肌表，则恶寒，自汗；在分肉，则麻木浮肿，其重如山，不利转侧，腰膝肿，筋骨痛，小溲秘，大便溏。"《医门法律•热湿暑三气门》也说："人身阳盛则轻娇，湿盛则身著，乃至身重如山，百脉痛楚，不能转侧。"均论述了湿邪阻滞经气而引起身体酸重疼痛的病机。治宜祛风散寒，除湿通络。方选《内外伤辨惑论》羌活胜湿汤（羌活、独活、防风、藁本、川芎、蔓荆子、甘草）。

1.2.4 Loss of Moistening due to Scant Liquid

The lung governs diffusion. This means that lung qì has the function of promoting the movement of defense qì and of the fluids. Thereby, it distributes the essence of grain and water through the entire body and warms and moistens the interstices of the flesh, the skin, and body hair. The chapter, "Understanding Qì" in the *Líng Shū* ("The Magic Pivot") states: "When the upper burner effuses, it diffuses the flavor of the five grains and warms the skin, fills the body, and moisturizes the body hair, just like a misting by fog or dew. This refers to qì." When this quotation states that "the upper burner effuses," this refers to the lung's functions of diffusing, distributing, and moistening.

When dryness-heat evil invades the lung, it produces two effects: On the one hand, lung-defense loses its ability to diffuse and qì fails to distribute liquid, which can cause loss of moistening due to scant liquid. On the other hand, dryness by its nature is dry and astringent, so it easily absorbs water. When heat evil blazes inside, it can easily damage the fluids. This can also cause loss of moistening due to scant liquid. As the bowels and viscera, offices and orifices, flesh, skin, and body hair are deprived of nourishment, this in turn causes such symptoms as dryness in the mouth, throat, nose, lips, tongue, and skin, parched dry hair, dry cough with scant phlegm, and shortened and reduced urination and dry and reduced defecation.

The chapter, "Concurrent Patterns in Cold Damage" in the *Chóng Dìng Tōng Sú Shāng Hán Lùn* ("Revised Popular On Cold Damage") states:

> "When warm dryness damages the lung, it initially results in headache and generalized heat effusion, dry cough without phlegm, and then in expectoration of phlegm that is mostly thin and sticky, qì counterflow and panting, sore dry throat, dry nose and lips, fullness in the chest, rib-side pain, heart vexation, thirst in the mouth, and a tongue with a dry thin white fur and redness on both sides and the tip."

The chapter,"Damage from Dryness" in the *Yī Biǎn* ("Lancing Stones of Medicine") also states:

> "On the outside, it manifests in chapped, raw, and dry skin; in the upper body, in a parched and dry nose and throat; in the lower body, in desiccated and astringed stool and urine; in the extremities, in wilting, weakness, and lack of strength; in the vessels in roughness, stagnation, vacuity, and debilitation."

Both these quotations describe all the symptoms of dryness that result from dryness evil damaging liquid and causing loss of moistening due to scant liquid.

This condition is treated by clearing and diffusing dryness-heat, and by engendering liquid and moistening the lung. The recommended formula is *shā shēn mài dōng tāng* (Adenophora/glehnia and Ophiopogon Decoction) from the *Wēn Bìng Tiáo Bian* ("Systematized Identification of Warm Diseases").

Shā Shēn Mài Dōng Tāng 沙参麦冬汤 (Adenophora/glehnia and Ophiopogon Decoction)
shā shēn 沙参 (Adenophorae seu Glehniae Radix, adenophora/glehnia)
mài mén dōng 麦门冬(Ophiopogonis Radix, ophiopogon)
sāng yè 桑叶 (Mori Folium, mulberry leaf)
yù zhú 玉竹 (Polygonati Odorati Rhizoma, Solomon's seal)
bái biǎn dòu 白扁豆 (Lablab Semen Album, lablab)
tiān huā fěn 天花粉 (Trichosanthis Radix, trichosanthes root)
gān cǎo 甘草 (Glycyrrhizae Radix, licorice)

津少失濡

肺主宣发，是指肺气有推动卫气、津液以及水谷精微输布全身，以温润肌腠皮毛的作用。《灵枢•决气篇》曰: "上焦开发，宣五谷味，熏肤、充身、泽毛，如雾露之溉，是谓气。" 所谓上焦开发，就是指肺的宣发、输布、濡润作用。燥热之邪犯肺，一方面，肺卫失宣，气不布津，可致津少失濡。另一方面，燥性干涩，易吸收水分；邪热炎炽，易耗伤津液，均可导致津少失濡，脏腑、官窍、肌肉、皮毛失养，引起口、咽、鼻、唇、舌、皮肤干燥、毛发焦枯、干咳少痰，二便短少等症。如《重订通俗伤寒论•伤寒兼证》曰: "温燥伤肺，初起头疼身热，干咳无痰，即咯痰多稀而黏，气逆而喘，咽喉干痛，鼻干唇燥，胸满胁疼，心烦口渴，舌苔白薄而燥，边尖俱红。" 《医碥•伤燥》又曰: "在外则皮肤皴揭枯涩，在上则鼻咽焦干，在下则二便涸涩，在手足则痿弱无力，在脉则涩滞虚衰。" 均论述燥邪伤津，津少失濡可引起各种干燥的症状。治宜清宣燥热，生津润肺。方选《温病条辨》沙参麦冬汤（沙参、麦冬、玉竹、花粉、扁豆、桑叶、甘草）。

1.2.5. Water Qì Flooding and Spilling

The lung is the upper source of water; lung qì has the function of regulating the waterways. When evil qì of wind, cold, dampness, heat, etc., assails from the outside, lung-defense loses its ability to diffuse. Qì and liquid are not distributed and therefore unable to enter the bowels and viscera on the inside or stray into the skin on the outside. In the lower body, the lung is unable to ensure regulated flow through the waterways, and water qì floods. It collects in the interior of the skin and causes generalized water swelling, with tightly stretched skin, joint pain, and wind water.

The chapter, "Pulse Symptoms and Treatments of Water Qì Disease" in the *Jīn Guì Yào Lüe* ("Essential Prescriptions of the Golden Coffer") explains: "Wind water manifests in swelling all over the whole body, a floating pulse, thirst, and spontaneous and continuous sweating without great heat. *Yuè bì tāng* (Spleen-Effusing Decoction) governs it." The *Sù Wèn* ("Plain Questions"), "Treatise on Points for Water and Heat" confirms that people in the past were familiar with the notions that wind water "is rooted in the kidney" and is caused by kidney vacuity sweating and contraction of wind. An analysis of *yuè bì tāng* (Spleen-Effusing Decoction) shows that the action of *má huáng* (Ephedrae Herba) to diffuse the lung and move water causes wind water to be dispersed. Thus we know that lung-defense failing to diffuse and flooding of water qì is an important pathomechanism for inducing wind water.

The "General Introduction to Swelling and Distention" in the *Zhèng Yīn Mài Zhì* ("Pathoconditions: Causes, Pulses, and Treatments") also explains:

> "In all cases of cold-related generalized swelling, the cause is a constitutional vacuity of exterior qì and constitutional heat of lung qì. Vacuity of the exterior results in easy entering of external evils; lung qì heat results in easy opening of the skin and body hair. When cold assails the fleshy exterior and becomes depressed instead of dispersing, it manifests in heat effusion with generalized swelling."

This quotation describes the pathomechanism by which an assault of wind-cold evil on the fleshy exterior prevents lung-defense from diffusing and the fluids from being distributed, so that they flood all over the body and cause water swelling.

This condition is treated by coursing wind and resolving the exterior, and by diffusing the lung and moving water. The recommended formula is *yuè bì jiā zhú tāng* (Spleen-Effusing Decoction Plus White Atractylodes) from the *Jīn Guì Yào Lüe* ("Essential Prescriptions of the Golden Coffer").

Yuè Bì Jiā Zhú Tāng 越婢汤 (Spleen-Effusing Decoction Plus White Atractylodes)
má huáng 麻黄 (Ephedrae Herba, ephedra)
shí gāo 石膏 (Gypsum Fibrosum, gypsum)
bái zhú 白朮 (Atractylodis Macrocephalae Rhizoma, white atractylodes)
shēng jiāng 生姜 (Zingiberis Rhizoma Recens, fresh ginger)
dà zǎo 大枣 (Jujubae Fructus, jujube)
gān cǎo 甘草 (Glycyrrhizae Radix, licorice)

To summarize, either evil qì of the six excesses entering through the mouth, nose, skin, and body hair, or phlegm turbidity and water-damp arising internally can depress lung qì and thereby impair diffusion. When the lung fails to diffuse, lung qì is unable to flow freely to the upper body. The body is unable to exhale qì outward, turbid qì remains inside, breathing is inhibited, and fullness and oppression in the chest occurs. The accumulating turbid qì is unable to descend and instead ascends counterflow. This ultimately leads to inhibited breathing with such symptoms as cough, counterflow, and asthma.

水气泛溢

肺为水之上源，肺气有通调水道的作用。风、寒、湿、热等邪气外袭，肺卫失宣，气津不布，内不得入于脏腑，外不得越于皮肤，下不能通行水道，水气泛溢，停留皮里，全身水肿、皮肤绷急、骨节疼痛、发为风水。《金匮要略•水气病脉证并治》说: “风水，一身悉肿，脉浮而渴，续自汗出，无大热，越婢汤主之”。前人有风水“本之于肾”（《素问•水热穴论》，为肾虚汗出受风而致之说。根据越婢汤以麻黄宣肺行水使风水得消来分析，肺卫失宣，水气泛溢应当为诱发风水的重要病机。《症因脉治•肿胀总论》又说: “凡寒身肿之因: 表气素虚，肺气素热，表虚则外邪易入，肺气热则皮毛易开，寒袭于肌表，郁而不散，则发热身肿之症作矣。”论述风寒之邪袭于肌表，肺卫失宣，水津失布，泛溢全身而成水肿的病机。治宜疏风解表，宣肺行水。方选《金匮要略》越婢加术汤（麻黄、石膏、白术、生姜、大枣、甘草）。

总之，六淫邪气从口鼻皮毛而入，痰浊水湿病理产物从内而生，均会遏郁肺气，导致宣发失职。肺失宣发，肺气不能上通，呼气不出，浊气存内，呼吸失畅，胸中满闷。积存之浊气不能下降，逆而向上，最终导致呼吸不利，引起咳逆气喘等症。

Literature Review of Impaired Diffusion of Lung Defense

📖 *Sù Wèn* (“Plain Questions”), “Treatise on Bone Hollow”

> “Wind entering from the outside causes quivering with cold, sweating, headache, generalized heaviness, and aversion to cold.”

This quotation describes the pathomechanism by which wind evil invading the lung prevents lung-defense from diffusing, which leads to loosening of the interstices and sweating with aversion to cold.

📖 *Sù Wèn* ("Plain Questions"), "Treatise on Needling Heat"

> "Lung heat disease manifests first in sudden shivering reversal, raised body hair, aversion to wind and cold, yellow tongue fur, and generalized heat effusion. When the heat struggles, it causes panting and cough, wandering pain in the anterior chest and back, inability to breathe deeply, unbearable headache, sweating, and cold."

This is the earliest text to describe wind-heat invading the lung and lung-defense failing to diffuse, manifesting in such symptoms as heat effusion, aversion to cold, and sweating.

📖 *Jīn Guì Yào Lüè* ("Essential Prescriptions of the Golden Coffer"), "Pulse Symptoms and Treatments of Water Qì Disease"

> "In wind water, the pulse is naturally floating, and the external signs are joint pain and aversion to wind. When the inch opening pulse is sunken and slippery, and there is water qì in the center, the head and face are swollen and enlarged, and there is heat, this is called 'wind water.' One sees slight swelling of the eye nest, as [in one] newly arisen from sleep; the neck pulse stirs, and there is frequent coughing. When you press the hands or feet, they pit but do not spring back. [All this constitutes] wind water."

This quotation describes the pathomechanical changes and clinical manifestations that result when evil qì assails from the outside, lung-defense loses its ability to diffuse, qì and liquid are not distributed, and water qì floods and collects in the interior of the skin, causing generalized water swelling.

📖 *Yī Mén Fǎ Lǜ* ("Axioms of Medicine"), "Section on Cough"

> "Cough that results from wind overwhelming the lung manifests in sweating, headache, and inhibition of phlegm-drool. Cough that results from fire overwhelming the lung manifests in rapid panting with congestion and counterflow, and in sniffle and spittle that contain blood. Cough that results from heat overwhelming the lung manifests in rapid panting with redness and tidal heat; in severe cases of heat exuberance in the center, in paradoxical cold in the four extremities; and when the heat shifts downward, in intolerable diarrhea. Cough that results from dryness overwhelming the lung results in dry skin and body hair, delicate sores that are damp and itchy, and constipation from adhering phlegm. Cough that results from cold overwhelming the lung manifests in aversion to cold without sweating, nasal congestion and generalized pain, heat effusion, and agitated vexation."

This quotation describes the particular pathomechanical changes and clinical manifestations that result when the evil qì of each of the six excesses (wind, fire, heat, dryness, cold, damp) invade the lung and prevent lung-defense from diffusing.

📖 *Zhèng Yīn Mài Zhì* ("Pathoconditions: Causes, Pulses, and Treatments"), "Dryness Damage Cough"

> "The signs of dryness damage cough are thirst and parched lips, heat vexation with taking fluids, phlegm that cannot be ejected, perhaps with strands of blood in it, redness in the stool and urine, and rapid panting and cough. These are the signs of dryness damage cough."

This quotation describes the clinical manifestations resulting when dampness evil invades the lung and damages liquid, so that it becomes scant and is not distributed, resulting in impaired nourishment to the lung, the offices and orifices, skin and flesh, and stool and urine.

📖 *Zhèng Yīn Mài Zhì* ("Pathoconditions: Causes, Pulses, and Treatments"), "Internal Damage Swelling"

> "Here is the cause of lung vacuity water swelling: Excessive taxation leads to a chronic vacuity of lung qì. The lung fails to command depuration and its power to downbear is impaired. Defense qì is congested and trapped, and construction qì is unable to follow. This results in the signs of swelling."

This quotation describes the pathomechanism by which lung-defense qì congestion and failure to diffuse can form water swelling.

文献评述

《素问•骨空论》曰："风从外入，令人振寒，汗出头痛，身重而寒。"论述风邪犯肺，肺卫失宣，可致肌腠疏松而汗出恶寒的病机。

《素问•刺热篇》云："肺热病者，先淅然厥，起毫毛，恶风寒，舌上黄，身热。热争，则喘咳，痛走胸膺背，不得大息，头痛不堪，汗出而寒。"最早描述了风热犯肺，肺卫失宣，可致发热、恶寒、汗出等症。

《金匮要略•水气病脉证并治》曰："风水，其脉自浮，外证骨节疼痛，恶风。…寸口脉沉滑者，中有水气，面目肿大，有热，名曰风水。视人之目窠上微肿，如蚕新卧起状，其颈脉动，时时咳，按其手足上。陷而不起者，风水。"阐述了邪气外袭，肺卫失宣，气津不布，水气泛溢，停留皮里，而成全身水肿的病机变化及临床表现。

《医门法律•咳嗽门》曰："风乘肺咳，汗出头痛，痰涎不利。火乘肺咳，喘急壅逆，涕唾见血。热乘肺咳，喘急而赤潮热，甚者热盛于中，四末反寒，热移于下，便泄无度。燥乘肺咳，皮毛干槁，细疮湿痒，痰胶便秘。寒乘肺咳，恶寒无汗，鼻塞身疼，发热躁烦。" 分别阐述风、火、热、燥、寒等六淫邪气犯肺，肺卫失宣所引起的病机变化及临床表现。

《症因脉治•伤燥咳嗽》曰:“伤燥咳嗽之症，口渴唇焦，烦热引饮，吐痰不出，或带血缕，二便带赤，喘急咳嗽，此伤燥咳嗽之症也。”阐述了燥邪犯肺伤津，津少失布，引起肺脏、官窍、肌肤、二便失养的临床表现。

《症因脉治•内伤肿胀》曰:“肺虚水肿之因:劳疫过度，肺气久虚，清肃之令不行，下降之权失职，卫气壅遏，营气不从，则肿症作矣。”阐述肺卫之气壅遏，失于宣散，可形成水肿的病机。

Summary of Impaired Diffusion of Lung Defense

1. Obstruction of Defense Qì
   Assault on the exterior by the six excesses:
      Defense failing to provide warmth: Aversion to cold.
      Defensive yáng depression in the exterior: Heat effusion.
2. Disharmony in the Interstices of the Flesh
   Interstices closed and blocked: Aversion to cold without sweating (cold governs contracture and tautness).
   Interstices open and discharging: Sweating and aversion to wind (wind by nature tends to cause opening and discharge). Generalized heat effusion with sweating (summerheat-heat steaming).
3. Inhibited Flow of Channel Qì
   Frequent stirring of wind evil:
      Channel qì block: Wandering pain in the head and body, joints, and flesh.
      Loss of nourishment in the channels: Deviated eyes and mouth, numbness of the skin, rigidity of the limbs, spasms of the extremities.
   Cold congealing and contracting: Headache and painful stiff nape; generalized aching and lumbar pain; coldness and pain in the joints; hypertonicity of the extremities (contracture and tautness).
   Dampness evil stagnating and causing heaviness: Head heavy as if swathed; generalized heaviness, encumbrance, and fatigue; soreness in the flesh and joints that is heavy and fixed.
4. Loss of Moistening Due to Scant Liquid
   Dry mouth, throat, lips, nose, and skin; parched dry hair; dry cough with scant phlegm; shortened and reduced urination and defecation.
5. Water Qì Flooding and Spilling
   Generalized water swelling, stretching and tension in the skin, joint pain.

肺卫失宣

卫气遏阻

六淫袭表

卫失温煦—恶寒。

卫阳郁表—发热。

肌腠失调

腠理闭塞—无汗恶寒（寒主收引）。

腠理开泄—汗出恶风（风性开泄）。身热汗出（暑热蒸腾）。

经气不利

风邪善动

闭塞经气—头身、关节、肌肉走痛。

经脉失养—口眼歪邪、肌肤麻木、肢体强直、手足痉挛。

寒凝收引—头项强痛、身疼腰痛、骨节冷痛。手足拘急（收引）。

湿邪滞重—头重如裹、身重困倦、肌肉、骨节酸痛、重着不移。

津少失濡

口咽唇鼻皮干燥、毛发焦枯、干咳少痰、二便短少。

水气泛溢

全身水肿、皮肤绷急、骨节疼痛。

Chapter Two

Impaired Depurative Downbearing

The lung is the "florid canopy." It is positioned in the upper burner and occupies the highest place there. Under normal circumstances, the lung's qì dynamic performs depuration and downbearing. When lung qì depurates and downbears, it absorbs clear qì, distributes the subtle essences downward, distributes water and essence to the four directions, and moves simultaneously in all five channels. Thereby it safeguards the uninhibited flow in the pathways of qì and in the waterways. It enables yáng qì to warm the five viscera, six bowels, four limbs, and hundred bones and allows them to be enriched by the fluids. At the same time, it is able to cleanse the lung connector and expel waste matter. As a result, all the viscera are naturally quiet.

External evils can assail the lung and prevent lung qì from diffusing. Alternatively, pathologic substances like water-damp, phlegm-rheum, or static blood can cause stagnation. Either of these will inhibit the flow in the qì pathways of the lung and thereby prevent depuration and downbearing of lung qì. This results in the pathomechanical changes of counterflow ascent of lung qì, breakdown of depurative downbearing, and block in the upper orifices.

肺失肃降

肺为"华盖"，位于上焦，居其高位，肺之气机应以清肃下降为顺。肺气肃降，吸收清气，下布精微，水精四布，五经并行，保证气道通畅、水道通调，使五脏六腑、四肢百骸得到阳气的温煦和津液的滋养，并能洁净肺系，排泄废物，而诸脏自安。外邪袭肺，肺气不宣，或因水湿痰饮瘀血等病理产物留滞，使肺之气道不畅，清肃之令不行，肺气失降，引起肺气上逆，肃降失职，上窍闭塞等病机变化。

2.1 Counterflow Ascent of Lung Qì

The lung governs depurative downbearing. Thereby it is able to make lung qì flow downward, safeguard the inhalation and absorption of clear qì from the natural environment, and cause it to be distributed throughout the entire body. The lung is the delicate viscus. As such, it likes clearness and purity and does not tolerate abnormal substances. As soon as it suffers an assault by external evil or stagnation of pathologic substances like water-damp, phlegm-rheum, or static blood, all of these can influence the ability of lung qì to bear downward to the lower body. When lung qì fails to downbear, upbearing and downbearing clash and ascend counterflow instead. This manifests in cough and counterflow, asthma, phlegm ejection, and other such symptoms of qì counterflow and upsurge.

The "Section on Cough" in the *Yī Fāng Lèi Jù* ("Collection of Classified Medical Formulas") states:

> "The reason for cough is that phlegm is obstructed in the chest and stomach duct and causes qì counterflow. Instead of descending, qì stirs the lung in surging attacks. How does this come about? I say that it is due to contraction of wind, cold, heat and dampness, and to static blood and collecting water, compounded by lung repletion or lung vacuity. All of these can congest phlegm and cause cough."

This quotation explains the pathomechanism by which a number of causes can congest lung qì and impair the lung's power to downbear, thereby forming the tendency to surge upward in counterflow.

Because the lung's loss of depurative downbearing is not an isolated pathomechanism but tends to be closely related to impaired diffusion of lung qì, it involves other issues besides lung qì counterflow ascent. These are treated it in the discussion of impaired diffusion of the lung.

肺气上逆

肺主肃降，能使肺气向下流通，保证吸纳自然界之清气，使之输布全身。肺为娇脏，喜清肃，不容异物，一旦受到外邪侵袭，或水湿痰饮瘀血等病理产物停留，均可影响肺气向下通降的功能。肺气不降，升降反作，逆而向上，表现咳逆气喘吐痰等一系列气逆冲上的症状。《医方类聚•咳嗽门》曰："所以咳嗽者，痰塞胸脘，气逆不下，冲击而动肺耳。然亦何以致此哉？曰感风伤冷，挟热受湿，瘀血停水，与夫肺实肺虚，皆能壅痰而发咳也。"说明各种原因壅塞肺气，肺失下降之权，则向形成会上冲逆的病机。由于肺失肃降不是一个单独的病机，常与肺气失宣密切相关，故涉及肺气上逆的其它内容，放入肺失宣降中讨论。

Literature Review of Counterflow Ascent of Lung Qì

📖 *Zhū Bìng Yuán Hòu Lùn* ("The Origin and Indicators of Disease"), "The Various Symptoms of Cough Disease; Symptoms of Cough with Qì Ascent"

> "Cough with qì ascent indicates a superabundance of lung qì. When the lung contracts cold, in mild cases it causes coughing. The lung governs qì, and when qì is superabundant, the result is panting and cough with qì ascent. This is related to the fact that evil has struck qì so that qì becomes congested and cannot diffuse. The result is superabundance, which is precisely the cause of cough and qì ascent. Its symptom is cough with qì ascent, profuse snivel and spittle, puffy swelling in the face and eyes, and qì counterflow."

This quotation describes how external evil invading the lung causes a superabundance of lung qì and inability to diffuse so that lung qì ascends counterflow, which can cause such signs of systemic lung disease as cough, panting, and qì counterflow.

文献评述

《诸病源候论•咳嗽病诸候•咳嗽上气候》：曰："夫咳嗽上气者，肺气有余也。肺感于寒，微则成咳嗽。肺主气，气有余则喘咳上气，此为邪搏于气，气壅不得宣发，是为有余，故咳嗽而上气也。其状咳嗽上气，多涕唾而面目胕肿，气逆也。"论述外邪犯肺，肺气有余，不得宣发，肺气上逆可引起咳喘气逆等多种肺系病证。

2.2 Breakdown of Depurative Downbearing

The lung occupies the highest place; it is often described as the florid canopy. When lung qì functions smoothly, it depurates and downbears. This depurative downbearing allows stomach qì to avoid abnormal counterflow ascent. At the same time it safeguards the downward movement of large intestinal qì and activates its normal function of conveyance. Thus it causes the qì dynamic of the stomach and intestine to move freely without obstruction. If external evil assails the lung and blocks lung qì, depuration is stopped, lung qì is unable to downbear, and large intestinal conveyance is impaired. Waste matter collects in the intestine and causes accumulation, stagnation, and stoppage in the large intestine. This results in stool that is bound, rough, and difficult to expel. When this condition progresses further to the point of intestinal qì stagnation, it manifests in abdominal pain and fullness, counterflow ascent of turbid qì, and other such symptoms.

The chapter, "Pulses of Stool and Urine Disease" in the *Mài Jué* ("Pulse Rhymes") states: "The lung pulse is floating and at the same time replete; the entrance to the throat is dry and damaged; defecation is difficult and rough; and the nose lacks a sense of smell." In the form of summary verses, this quotation describes concisely the pathomechanism by which lung qì failing to downbear can result in intestinal qì stagnation and bowel qì stoppage.

The chapter, "Yīn and Yáng Viscera and Bowels" in the *Shèn Zhāi Yí Shū* ("Shen-Zai's Legacy") points out even more clearly: "When turbid qì is located in the upper body, it fills up and congests lung qì. The lung is unable to carry out downbearing, and this causes fecal block."

The "Section on Urine and Stool" in the *Gŭ Jīn Tú Shū Jí Chéng Yī Bù Quán Lù Jīng Huá Běn* ("Grand Compendium of Books from the Past to the Present; Medical Section; Choice Selections from the Entire Record") quotes an explanation by Zhū Dān-Xī that discusses contraindications for freeing the stool:

> "When I look at the ancient formulas, those for freeing the stool all use ingredients that downbear qì. When lung qì fails to downbear, stool is passed only with difficulty. This is the reason for using medicinals like *xìng rén* (Armeniacae Semen), *zhǐ qiào* (*ké*) (Aurantii Fructus), *chén xiāng* (Aquilariae Lignum Resinatum), and *zhī zǐ* (Gardeniae Fructus)."

Yè Tiān-Shì further analyzed constipation in detail from the angle of impaired depurative downbearing of the lung, on the basis of numerous medical case histories. In his *Lín Zhèng Zhǐ Nán Yī Àn* ("A Clinical Guide with Case Histories"), there are three sections of case histories on intestinal impediment, lung impediment, and constipation, in which he repeatedly stressed the relationship between constipation and lung qì repletion block. He suggested that cold, heat, dryness, dampness, wind, and fire could all lead to lung qì blockage, stopped depuration, and impaired intestinal conveyance, thereby resulting in constipation.

In addition to describing rather comprehensively the disease causes and pathomechanisms of constipation on the basis of differentiating and treating the lung, he also advocated opening and downbearing lung qì in the upper burner to free the stool naturally. Consequently he stressed "upraising the orifices of the lung" as the fundamental principle for treating constipation. For example, in the chapter "Intestinal Impediment" in the *Lín Zhèng Zhǐ Nán Yī Àn* ("A Clinical Guide with Case Histories"), he explained:

> "The constipation associated with intestinal impediment is milder than that of dry hard bound stool that cannot be passed despite the urge to defecate; so the master treated it by merely opening and downbearing the upper burner and lung qì. This treatment caused the upper orifices to open and discharge, so that the lower orifices were spontaneously freed."

If phlegm-turbidity blocks the lung, it manifests in qì counterflow panting and cough, phlegm that is copious, white, and easy to expectorate, abdominal fullness and constipation, a white slimy tongue fur, and a stringlike pulse.

This condition is treated by drying dampness and transforming phlegm, and by downbearing qì and freeing the stool. The recommended formula is *sū zǐ jiàng qì tāng* (Perilla Seed Qì-Downbearing Decoction) from the *Tài Píng Huì Mín Hé Jì Jú Fāng* (Tài-Píng Imperial Grace Pharmacy Formulas) with the addition of *bīng láng* (Arecae Semen).

Sū Zǐ Jiàng Qì Tāng 苏子降气汤 (Perilla Seed Qì-Downbearing Decoction)

zǐ sū zǐ 紫苏子 (Perillae Fructus, perilla fruit)
qián hú 前胡 (Peucedani Radix, peucedanum)
hòu pò 厚朴 (Magnoliae Officinalis Cortex, officinal magnolia bark)
chén pí 陈皮 (Citri Reticulatae Pericarpium, tangerine peel)
bàn xià 半夏 (Pinelliae Rhizoma, pinellia)
ròu guì 肉桂 (Cinnamomi Cortex, cinnamon bark)
dāng guī 当归 (Angelicae Sinensis Radix, Chinese angelica)
shēng jiāng 生姜 (Zingiberis Rhizoma, fresh ginger Recens)
gān cǎo 甘草 (Glycyrrhizae Radix, licorice)
Plus:
bīng láng 槟榔 (Arecae Semen, areca)

If evil heat congests the lung and impairs the lung's depurative downbearing, you will see not only high fever, rough breathing, and cough and panting with thick yellow phlegm, but at the same time the combined signs of abdominal distention and fullness, pain that refuses pressure, constipation, and large intestinal dryness-heat. This condition is treated by clearing heat and draining the lung, and by downbearing qì and freeing the stool. For a formula, select *xuān bái chéng qì tāng* (White-Diffusing Qì-Coordinating Decoction) from the *Wēn Bìng Tiáo Bian* ("Systematized Identification of Warm Diseases").

Xuān Bái Chéng Qì Tāng 宣白承气汤
(White-Diffusing Qì-Coordinating Decoction)

shí gāo 石膏 (Gypsum Fibrosum, gypsum)
dà huáng 大黄 (Rhei Radix et Rhizoma, rhubarb)
xìng rén 杏仁 (Armeniacae Semen, apricot kernel)
guā lóu pí 栝楼皮（Trichosanthis Pericarpium, trichosanthes rind)

When the lung's depurative downbearing is impaired, it can influence the conveyance of stool in two ways: As described above, when depurative downbearing is stopped and lung qì is unable to downbear, this obstructs large intestinal conveyance and can lead to constipation. Conversely, if evil qì invades the lung and toxic heat causes distress, this can make the lung's depurative downbearing excessive. Evil toxin, together with water-damp, can squeeze lung qì to rush straight into the large intestine, where it wreaks havoc on conveyance. This results in the symptom of diarrhea and sloppy stool.

As we can see from diarrhea in children suffering from measles, for example, this is indeed caused by lung heat shifting to the large intestine. The "Heart Approach to Pox Papules in Rhyme" in the *Yī Zōng Jīn Jiàn* ("The Golden Mirror of Medicine") explains: "Diarrhea from measles means that toxic heat has passed into the intestines and stomach, where it has disordered conveyance. This causes abdominal pain with desire to defecate and stool that is sometimes red, sometimes white, and sometimes a combination of red and white." When the evil heat in measles congests the lung and cannot be outthrust, the force of the heat distresses the body internally. In spite of the fact that it surges upward in counterflow, it cannot be outthrust from there either. In this case, it invariably combines with the toxic evils of phlegm and heat and drain into the lower body. Forcing lung qì downward, this causes diarrhea.

This condition is treated by clearing the lung and draining heat, and by freeing the intestines and downbearing stagnation. The recommended formula is *qīng rè dǎo zhì tāng* (Clear Heat and Abduct Stagnation Decoction) from the *Yī Zōng Jīn Jiàn* ("The Golden Mirror of Medicine").

Qīng Rè Dǎo Zhì Tāng 清热导滞汤 (Clear Heat and Abduct Stagnation Decoction)
huáng qín 黄芩 (Scutellariae Radix, scutellaria)
huáng lián 黄连 (Coptidis Rhizoma, coptis)
lián qiào 连翘 (Forsythiae Fructus, forsythia)
niú bàng zǐ 牛蒡子 (Arctii Fructus, arctium)
shān zhā 山楂 (Crataegi Fructus, crataegus)
hòu pò 厚朴 (Magnoliae Officinalis Cortex, officinal magnolia bark)
qīng pí 陈皮 (Citri Reticulatae Pericarpium Viride, tangerine peel)
zhǐ qiào (*ké*) 枳壳 (Aurantii Fructus, bitter orange)
bīng láng 槟榔 (Arecae Semen, areca)
bái sháo 白芍 (Paeoniae Radix Alba, white peony)
dāng guī 当归 (Angelicae Sinensis Radix, Chinese angelica)
gān cǎo 甘草 (Glycyrrhizae Radix, licorice)

In addition, an external contraction of the evil qì of the six excesses can prevent lung-defense from diffusing and, as the evil distresses the large intestine, derange conveyance. This can cause dysentery with abdominal urgency and rectal heaviness. Yù Jiā recommended the method of treating dysentery by opening and raising lung qì, like hauling a boat upstream. This is formulated on the basis of this pathomechanism of excessive depurative downbearing by lung qì.

This conditionis treated by diffusing lung qì and by eliminating dampness and checking diarrhea. The recommended formula is *huó rén bài dú sǎn* (Life Saving Toxin-Vanquishing Powder) from the *Yī Mén Fǎ Lǜ* ("Axioms of Medicine").

Huó Rén Bài Dú Sǎn 败毒散 (Life Saving Toxin-Vanquishing Powder)
qiāng huó 羌活 (Notopterygii Rhizoma et Radix, notopterygium)
dú huó 独活 (Angelicae Pubescentis Radix, pubescent angelica)
qián hú 前胡 (Peucedani Radix, peucedanum)
chái hú 柴胡 (Bupleuri Radix, bupleurum)
chuān xiōng 川芎 (Chuanxiong Rhizoma, chuanxiong)
zhǐ qiào (*ké*) 枳壳 (Aurantii Fructus, bitter orange)
fú líng 茯苓 (Poria, poria)
rén shēn 人参 (Ginseng Radix, ginseng)
gān cǎo 甘草 (Glycyrrhizae Radix, licorice)

肃降失职

肺居高位，为华盖之脏，肺气以肃降为顺。肺气肃降，可使胃气无上逆之变，同时能保证大肠之气下行，发挥正常的传导功能，使胃肠气机畅行无阻。若邪气袭肺，肺气闭塞，清肃之令不行，肺气不能下降，大肠传导失职，糟粕停留肠间，大肠积滞不通，则引起大便秘结，艰涩难排。进而肠中气滞，出现腹痛腹满、浊气上逆等症。《脉诀•大小便病脉》云："肺脉浮兼实，咽门燥又伤，大便难且涩，鼻内乏馨香。"用歌括形式，简明扼要地阐述了肺气不能下降，可致肠道气滞，腑气不通的病机。《慎斋遗书•阴阳脏腑》更明白指出："浊气在上，则填塞肺气，肺不能行下降之令，故大便闭。"《医部全录•大小便门》引朱丹溪论通大便禁忌说："予观古方，通大便皆用降气之品，盖肺气不降，则大便难传送，用杏仁、枳壳、沉香、栀子等是也。" 叶天士更以大量医案从肺失肃降的角度对便秘进行深入探讨，他在《临证指南医案》肠痹、肺痹、便闭等三篇医案中反复提到大便闭结与肺气闭实的关系，认为寒、热、燥、湿、风、火等原因均可导致肺气闭塞，清肃不行，肠道传导失司而引起便秘，不仅较为全面阐述便秘从肺辨治的病因、病机，而且认为开降上焦肺气，则大便自通，从而提出“升提肺窍”作为治疗便秘的基本法则。如《临证指南医案•肠痹》说：“盖肠痹之便闭，较之燥屎坚结欲便不通者稍缓，故先生但开降上焦肺气，上窍开泄，下窍自通。”若痰浊闭肺，咳喘气逆，痰多色白易咯，腹满便秘，苔白厚腻，脉弦。治宜燥湿化痰，降气通便。方选《和剂局方》苏子降气汤（苏子、前胡、厚朴、陈皮、半夏、肉桂、当归、生姜、甘草）加槟榔。

若邪热壅肺，肺失肃降，在高热气粗，咳喘痰黄稠的同时，兼见腹部胀满，疼痛拒按，大便秘结，大肠燥热互结之证。治宜清热泻肺，降气通便。方选《温病条辨》宣白承气汤（生石膏、大黄、杏仁、括蒌皮）。

肺失肃降对大便传导功能的影响存在双向调节作用。如上所述，肃降不行，肺气不能下降，大肠传导阻滞，可致大便秘结。若邪气犯肺，毒热逼迫，可使肺气肃降太过，邪毒与水湿夹肺气直迫大肠，使之传导紊乱，引起腹泄便溏之症。如小儿麻疹所见泄泻，即是肺热移于大肠所成。《医宗金鉴•痘疹心法要诀》说：“麻疹泻泄，乃毒热移入肠胃，使传化失常也。有腹痛欲解，或赤或白，或赤白相兼者。”麻疹毒热壅肺，不得外透，热势内迫，虽向上冲逆，亦不能外透，势必夹杂痰热毒邪，向下排泻，逼迫肺气下降而成泻泄。治宜清肺泻热，通肠导滞。方选《医宗金鉴》清热导滞汤（黄芩、黄连、连翘、牛蒡子、山楂、厚朴、青皮、枳壳、槟榔、白芍、当归、甘草）. 此外，外感六淫邪气，肺卫失宣，邪迫大肠，传导失调可引起里急后重的下痢证。喻嘉言开提肺气，逆流挽舟而治疗痢疾之法，就是根据肺气肃降太过的病机而制定。治宜升宣肺气，除湿止泻。方选《医门法律》活人败毒散（羌活、独活、前胡、柴胡、川芎、枳壳、茯苓、人参、甘草）。

Literature Review of Breakdown of Depurative Downbearing

📖 *Zhōng Zàng Jīng* (“Central Treasury Canon”), “Discussing the Pulses and Patterns of Vacuity and Repletion, Cold and Heat, Life and Death, and Favorable and Unfavorable Shifts in Large Intestine Disease”

“The large intestine is the bowel of the lung. It trumpets conveyance[1] and oversees the granary. When lung disease is not halted, it can pass to the

[1] Author’s note: The use of the word “trumpets” suggests that the lung is in charge of issuing and implementing commands for the whole body.

> large intestine. The hand yáng brightness is its channel. Coldness results in diarrhea, warmth in constipation…Again, heat repletion manifests in painful distention and fecal stoppage."

This quotation suggests that when the evil qì of repletion heat invades the lung, it can lead to fecal stoppage. Thus it illustrates from the angle of pathology how a breakdown of the lung's depurative downbearing can cause constipation.

🕮 *Lín Zhèng Zhǐ Nán Yī Àn* ("A Clinical Guide with Case Histories"), "Fecal Block," Jīn's case history

> "In a case of damp-heat in the channels, a previous physician had failed to treat in accordance with the symptoms and had subsequently allowed the condition to deteriorate into generalized qì obstruction. The evil was scattered all over, causing congestion, swelling, and redness. Initially the damp-heat had caused diarrhea, but had now resulted in orifice block, to the point of fecal and urinary stoppage. Nevertheless, by rectifying lung qì I was able to diffuse the evil. For this case of damp-heat with lung qì failing to downbear, I used *wěi jīng tāng* (Phragmites Stem Decoction), but left out *guī bǎn* (Testudinis Plastrum) and added *huá shí* (Talcum), *tōng cǎo* (Tetrapanacis Medulla), and *xī guā* (Citrulli Fructus)."

Huà Xiù summed up this treatment method in his commentary:

> "If damp-heat damages qì and obstructs the channels and bowels, then you rectify lung qì by opening and downbearing it."

This illustrates how damp-heat invading the lung, followed by lung qì depression block and breakdown of depurative downbearing, can lead to constipation. Furthermore, it emphasizes the treatment principle of opening and downbearing lung qì.

🕮 *Xuè Zhèng Lùn* ("On Blood Patterns"), "Fecal Block"

> "The lung and the large intestine stand in an exterior-interior relationship. When the lung transmits heat to the large intestine, when lung liquid fails to moisten, or when lung qì fails to downbear, the result is bound stool."

This indicates how lung heat damaging liquid can cause reduced liquid and loss of moistening, impaired depurative downbearing by the lung, and lung qì failing to propel, which all result in constipation.

🕮 *Shí Shì Mì Lù* ("Secret Records from the Stone Chamber"), "Dry Bound Stool"

> "People assume that bound stool is caused by severe dryness in the large intestine. Who is aware that it is related to dryness in lung qì? When the lung is dry, then depurating qì is unable to move downwards into the large intestine. In that case, the water in the kidney channel is barely sufficient to take care of itself. How could it also flow to moisten the little side streams?"

This describes how liquid damage from dryness-heat and impaired depurative downbearing by the lung can lead to constipation.

📖 *Yī Mén Fǎ Lǜ* ("Axioms of Medicine"), "Section on Cough"

> "Cough that results from wind overcoming the lung manifests in sweating, headache, and inhibited phlegm-drool. Cough that results from fire overcoming the lung manifests in rapid panting with congestion and counterflow, and in sniffle and spittle that contain blood. Cough that results from heat overcoming the lung manifests in rapid panting with redness and tidal heat; in severe cases of heat exuberance in the center, in paradoxical cold in the four extremities; and when the heat shifts downward, in intolerable diarrhea."

This describes the pathomechanism by which lung heat exuberance and excessive depurative downbearing can lead to incessant diarrhea when the heat shifts into the large intestine.

文献评述

《中藏经•论大肠虚实寒热生死逆顺脉证》曰: "大肠者，肺之腑也，为传送之司号，监仓之官。肺病不已，则传入大肠，手阳明是其经也。寒则泄，热则结，…又实热证胀满，而大便不通也。" 认为实热邪气犯肺可引起大便不通，从病理上阐明肺失肃降可致大便秘结。

《临证指南医案•便闭》金氏病案曰: "湿热在经，医不对症，遂令一身气阻，邪势散漫，壅肿赤块，初因湿热为泄泻，今则窍闭，致二便不通，但理肺气，邪可宣通。湿热肺气不降，苇茎汤去瓜瓣加滑石、通草、西瓜翠衣。" 华岫云在按语时归纳其治法云: "若湿热伤气，阻遏经腑者，则理肺气以开降之。" 阐明湿热犯肺，肺气闭郁，肃降失职，可致便秘，并提出开降肺气的治疗大法。

《血证论•便闭》曰: "肺与大肠相表里，肺遗热于大肠则便结，肺津不润则便结，肺气不降则便结。" 指出肺热伤津，津少失滋，肺失肃降，肺气失于推动，可致便秘。

《石室密录•大便燥结》云: "大便秘结者，人以为大肠燥甚，谁知是肺气燥乎？肺燥则清肃之气，不能下行于大肠，而肾经之水，仅足以自顾，又何能旁流以润溪涧哉？" 论述燥热津伤，肺失肃降，可致大便秘结。

《医门法律•咳嗽门》曰: "风乘肺咳，汗出头痛，痰涎不利。火乘肺咳，喘急壅逆，涕唾见血。热乘肺咳，喘急而赤潮热，甚者热盛于中，四末反寒，热移于下，便泄无度。" 阐述了肺热亢盛，肃降太过，热移大肠，可致腹泻下利不止的病机。

2.3 Block in the Upper Orifices

In normal physiological conditions, lung qì performs depurative downbearing, the fluids are transported down into the bladder, and the elimination of urine is regular. If external evil blocks the lung or if phlegm-heat obstructs the lung, evil heat damages the lung and exuberant heat damages liquid. When lung-metal is affected by dryness-heat, lung qì is unable to perform depurative downbearing, the fluids cannot be transported down to the bladder, and qì transformation fails. This causes dribbling urinary block.

In (*Dān Xī Xīn Fǎ* ("Dān Xī's Heart-Approach"), "Urinary Dribbling and Block")," Zhū Dān-Xī explained:

> "The lung is the upper burner; the bladder is the lower burner. When the upper burner is blocked, the lower burner becomes congested… It is like a utensil for dripping water: the upper orifice must be open for water to come out of the lower orifice."

The chapter, "Dribbling Urinary Block" in the *Jǐng Yuè Quán Shū* ("Jǐng-Yuè's Complete Compendium"), "Schema of Miscellaneous Patterns" also states:

> "In all patterns of qì repletion and the like, there is no better treatment than ejection. This is like a utensil for dripping water: If the upper orifice is blocked, the lower orifice is also stopped. If you open the upper orifice, it invariably frees the lower orifice. When you have upbearing, you have downbearing; when you don't have upbearing, then you also lack downbearing. This is the reason behind the dynamic of rectification."

This source illustrates the pathomechanism by which impaired depurative downbearing and block in the upper orifices causes urinary stoppage, from the perspective of the upbearing and downbearing of the qì dynamic. For treatment, the text recommends ejection to free urination, suggesting that when the upper orifices are freed, the lower orifices discharge on their own. Wú Jū also advocated the method of "opening the upper sluice, transforming lung qì, and diffusing the upper body, to disinhibit the lower body," when discussing the treatment of dribbling urinary block.

This condition is treated by lifting the pot and removing the lid, and by diffusing above and disinhibiting below. The appropriate formula is *èr chén tāng* (Two Matured Ingredients Decoction) with the addition of *mù tōng* (Akebiae Trifoliatae Caulis) and *xiāng fù* (Cyperi Rhizoma), to "lift qì and by making qì rise, make water descend naturally (*Dān Xī Xīn Fǎ* ("Dān Xī's Heart-Approach"), "Urinary Stoppage")."

Èr Chén Tāng 二陈汤 (Two Matured Ingredients Decoction)
bàn xià 半夏 (Pinelliae Rhizoma, pinellia) *fú líng* 茯苓 (Poria, poria) *chén pí* 陈皮 (Citri Reticulatae Pericarpium, tangerine peel) Plus: *mù tōng* 木通 (Akebiae Trifoliatae Caulis, trifoliate akebia) *xiāng fù* 香附 (Cyperi Rhizoma, cyperus)

If the lung suffers from exuberant heat, it loses its ability to perform depurative downbearing, and urination stops. This condition is treated by clearing the lung and draining heat, and by freeing urine. Ordinarily, the recommended formula is *qīng fèi yǐn* (Lung-Clearing Beverage) from the *Zhèng Zhì Huì Bǔ* ("Combined Supplements to Patterns and Treatment") with modifications.

Qīng Fèi Yǐn 清肺饮 (Lung-Clearing Beverage)
huáng qín 黄芩 (Scutellariae Radix, scutellaria) *zhī zǐ* 栀子 (Gardeniae Fructus, gardenia) *sāng bái pí* 桑白皮 (Mori Cortex, mulberry root bark) *fú líng* 茯苓 (Poria, poria) *mài mén dōng* 麦门冬 (Ophiopogonis Radix, ophiopogon) *mù tōng* 木通 (Akebiae Trifoliatae Caulis, trifoliate akebia) *chē qián zǐ* 车前子 (Plantaginis Semen, plantago seed)

In addition, when the lung's depurative downbearing is impaired, metal fails to restrain wood. This can lead to the pathomechanism of wood fire tormenting metal. A rather early reference to this pathomechanism comes from Lǐ Dōng-Yuán who explained the following in the chapter, "Dampness Damage in the Fall Causing Cough in Winter" in his *Dōng Yuán Shí Shū* ("Dong-Yuan's Ten Books"):

> "When the lung is deficient in autumn, the overcome phase (i.e. wood) moves frenetically. This means that fire is able to flame upward and overcome metal. When heart fire torments metal, lung qì moves counterflow and causes cough. The overcoming phase then rebels against it, and wood qì therefore moves upward. Wood and fire have the same virtues; they stir and do not rest."

Thus he was the first to state how heart fire damaging the lung makes lung qì ascend counterflow and stops depurative downbearing, resulting in the pathomechanism of liver qì rebelling.

Subsequently, the chapter, "Liver Channel Cough" in the *Zhèng Yīn Mài Zhì* ("Pathoconditions: Causes, Pulses, and Treatments") stated: "The cause of liver channel cough is wood qì depression, intermittent stirring of liver fire, and fire exuberance tormenting metal. This results in cough and panting." The author thus pointed out that liver fire invading the lung can cause cough and panting. In this context, he also emphasized that hyperactive wood tormenting metal ought to include the pathomechanism of lung qì losing control and wood rebelling against metal.

Táng Róng-Chuān was the first to describe this pathomechanism explicitly. In the "Treatise on the Pathomechanisms of the Viscera and Bowels" in the *Xuè Zhèng Lùn* ("On Blood Patterns, he explained: "When metal fails to restrain wood, liver fire is effulgent, and therefore fire torments metal. This results in steaming heat effusion, panting and cough, blood ejection, and consumption occurring simultaneously."

The reason for this is that the lung governs depurative downbearing and is cool by nature. The liver governs upbearing and effusing and also holds the ministerial fire. When lung qì depurates, it can prevent liver-wood and the ministerial fire from becoming excessive so that they engage in upbearing and effusing according to their nature. This means that metal is able to restrain wood, that lung qì depurates and moves downward, and that liver qì is harmonized. But when depurative downbearing of lung qì breaks down, liver wood is without restraint and upbears and effuses excessively. As a result, wood and fire rebel against lung-metal. This manifests in such symptoms as dizziness and headache, distention and pain in the chest and rib-sides, cough with counterflow and dry throat, and ejection of thick yellow phlegm.

This condition is treated by clearing the lung and draining fire, and by calming the liver and repressing wood. The recommended formula is *xiè bái sǎn* (White-Draining Powder) from the *Xiǎo Ér Yào Zhèng Zhí Jué* ("Key to Diagnosis and Treatment of Children's Diseases") in combination with *dài gé sǎn* (Indigo and Clamshell Powder).

Xiè Bái Sǎn 泻白散 (White-Draining Powder)
with *Dài Gé Sǎn* 黛蛤散 (Indigo and Clamshell Powder)

sāng bái pí 桑白皮 (Mori Cortex, mulberry root bark)
dì gǔ pí 地骨皮 (Lycii Cortex, lycium root bark)
jīng mǐ 粳米 (Oryzae Semen, non-glutinous rice)
gān cǎo 甘草 (Glycyrrhizae Radix, licorice)
Plus:
qīng dài 青黛 (Indigo Naturalis, indigo)
hǎi gé qiào (*ké*) 海蛤壳 (Meretricis seu Cyclinae Concha, clamshell)

上窍闭塞

正常生理状态下，肺气肃降，水液下输膀胱，小便排泄正常。若外邪闭肺或痰热阻肺，肺为邪热所伤，热盛津伤，肺金燥热，肺气不能肃降，津液不能下输膀胱，气化无权，发为癃闭。朱丹溪说："肺为上焦，膀胱为下焦，上焦闭则下焦塞...如滴水之器，必上窍通而后下窍之水出焉"（《丹溪纂要•淋闭》）。《景岳全书•杂证谟•癃闭》也曰："凡气实等证，无如吐之妙者，譬之滴水之器，闭其上窍，则下窍不通。开其上窍，则下窍必利。盖有升则有降，无升则无降，此理势之使然也。"从气机升降的角度，阐明肺失肃降，上窍闭塞，而小便不通的病机。治用吐法以通小便，取其上窍通，下窍自出之意。吴鞠通治疗癃闭也提出"启上闸，化肺气，宣上则利下"的治法。治宜提壶揭盖，宣上利下。方选二陈汤加木通、香附，"以提其气，气升则水自降下。"《丹溪心法•小便不通》。若肺热壅盛，失于肃降而小便不通，当清肺泻热，通利小便。常用《证治汇补》清肺饮（黄芩、栀子、桑白皮、茯苓、麦冬、木通、车前子）加减。

此外，肺失肃降，金不制木，可引起木火刑金的病机。较早提出这一病机的是李东垣，他在《东垣十书•秋伤于湿冬生咳嗽》曰：中说："秋令不及，所胜妄行，故火得以炎上而克金，心火既刑于肺，故肺气逆而为咳。所不胜者侮之，故木气上行，与火同德，动而不息也。"先言心火伤肺，肺气上逆，肃降不行，引出肝气反侮的病机。其后《症因脉治•肝经咳嗽》云："肝经咳嗽之因，木气怫郁，肝火时动，火盛刑金，则为咳喘。"提出肝火犯肺可致咳喘，这里强调木旺刑金，理当包含肺气失制，木反侮金的病机。直到唐容川，才明确地对这一病机作出论述。《血证论•脏腑病机论》说："金不制木，则肝火旺，火盛刑金，则蒸热，喘咳，吐血，痨瘵并作。"这是因为肺主肃降，其性清凉。肝主升发，含有相火。肺气清肃，可防止肝木相火太过，以遂其升发之性。即金能制木，肺气清肃下行，肝气得以调和。肺气肃降失职，肝木无制，升发太过，则木火反侮肺金，常见头晕头痛，胸胁胀痛，咳逆咽干，吐痰黄稠等症。治宜清肺泻火，平肝抑木。方选《小儿药证直诀》泻白散（桑白皮、地骨皮、粳米、甘草）合黛蛤散（青黛、海蛤壳）。

Literature Review of Block in the Upper Orifices

📖 *Xuè Zhèng Lùn* ("On Blood Patterns"), "Treatise on the Pathomechanisms of the Viscera and Bowels"

"The urinary bladder is known as the greater yáng channel. It is called yáng within water, and it reaches out with defense qì to the outer body.

> Thus it is really the greatest among all yáng. External contractions result in damage to defense yáng, and in heat effusion and aversion to cold...The skin and body hair are connected to the lung, and the lung is moreover the upper source of water. Therefore, to promote sweating, you must treat the lung, and to disinhibit water, you must also treat the lung."

This quotation discusses in passing that the urinary bladder is greater yáng and governs the exterior and that the lung is related to the skin and body hair. It also describes how evil invading the lung causes blockage of the upper orifices, lack of clarity in the upper origin, and inhibited urination. Therefore, to promote sweating, you should treat the lung; to disinhibit water, you should also treat the lung. By opening the upper orifices, you will unstop the lower orifices.

🕮 *Zhèng Zhì Huì Bǔ* ("Combined Supplements to Patterns and Treatment"), "Dribbling Urinary Block"

> "The qì in the entire body is connected to the lung. When the lung is clear, qì moves; when the lung is turbid, qì congests. Therefore, urinary stoppage is for the most part caused by lung qì failing to diffuse. It is appropriate to treat this primarily by clearing metal and downbearing qì."

This quotation further stresses the pathomechanism and treatment method for inhibited urination caused by lung turbidity with qì congestion, loss of depurative downbearing, and block in the upper orifices.

🕮 *Yī Biǎn* ("Lancing Stones of Medicine"), "Coughing of Blood"

> "When fire torments metal, the lung's lobes become dry and wrinkled. This causes them to itch. Itching results in cough, which does not necessarily produce phlegm. Therefore it is called dry cough. Profuse coughing results in damage to the lung network vessels. This causes bleeding."

This quotation describes the pathomechanism by which impaired depurative downbearing of the lung, and wood fire tormenting metal results in dry cough and ejection of blood.

🕮 *Zhī Yī Bì Biàn* ("Essential Differentiations in Medical Knowledge"), "Cough"

> "The lung belongs to metal, which is originally supposed to restrain wood. However, when liver qì is overly effulgent and not restrained by metal, it will turn around and rebel against metal. This impairs depuration of the lung and leads to incessant choking and coughing. This is called wood attacking and metal ringing."

Through the metaphor of wood tapping and metal ringing, this quotation illustrates the pathomechanism of impaired depuration by the lung, metal failing to restrain wood, and wood-fire tormenting metal.

文献评述

《血证论•脏腑病机论》曰: "膀胱称为太阳经，谓水中之阳，达于外以卫气，乃阳中之最大者也。外感则伤其卫阳，发热恶寒。…皮毛与肺合，肺又为水之上源，故发汗需治肺，利水亦需治肺。"通过论述膀胱为太阳主表，肺合皮毛而相互关联。阐述肺受邪侵，上窍闭塞，上源不清，小便不利时，可发汗治肺，利水治肺，开上窍而通下窍。

《证治汇补•癃闭》曰: "一身之气关于肺，肺清则气行，肺浊则气壅，故小便不通，由肺气不能宣布者居多，宜清金降气为主。"进一步强调，肺浊气壅，失于肃降，上窍闭塞，小便不通的病机和治法。

《医碥•咳嗽血》曰: "火刑金而肺叶干皱则痒，痒则咳，此不必有痰，故名干咳，咳多则肺络伤，而血出矣。"阐述了肺失肃降，木火刑金，引起干咳，咯血的病机。

《知医必辨•咳嗽》曰: "肺属金，原以制木，而肝气太旺，不受金制，反来侮金，致肺之清肃不行，而呛咳不已，所谓木击金鸣也。"以木叩金鸣的形象比喻，阐明肺失清肃，金不制木，木火刑金的病机。

Summary of Impaired Depurative Downbearing of the Lung

1. Counterflow Ascent of Lung Qì

   Cough, counterflow, panting (asthma).

2. Stopped Depurative Downbearing

   Breakdown of conveyance: Bound stool that is rough and difficult to expel. Intestinal qì stagnation, abdominal fullness and pain.

3. Excessive Depurative Downbearing

   Toxic heat distressing the lung: Heat distressing the large intestine: Diarrhea and sloppy stool

4. Blockage of the Upper Orifices

   Lung-metal dryness-heat: Liquid depletion in the urinary bladder: Dribbling urinary block.

肺失肃降

肺气上逆——咳逆气喘。

肃降不行——传导失职—大便秘结、艰涩难行。

肠中气滞，腹满腹痛。

肃降太过——毒热迫肺——热迫大肠——腹泻便溏。

上窍闭塞——肺金燥热——膀胱津亏——癃闭。

Chapter Three

Impaired Diffusion and Downbearing

Diffusion and depurative downbearing are the most basic aspects of the lung's physiological activity. They complement each other and thereby safeguard the normal performance of the many other physiological functions by the lung. When pathological changes occur, they can manifest singly as impaired diffusion by lung qì or as impaired downbearing by lung qì. Nevertheless, in the vast majority of cases, these affect each other and are impaired at the same time. This manifests as breakdown of diffusion and downbearing in the lung. The pathomechanical changes related to impaired diffusion and downbearing of the lung can be differentiated into three large categories: Qì dynamic disorders; non-distribution of the fluids; and qì and blood depression.

肺失宣降

肺的生理运动以宣发、肃降为基本形式。宣发肃降相辅相成，保证肺的多种生理功能正常进行。发生病理变化时，既可单独表现为肺气失宣，或肺气失降，但大多数情况下是相互影响，同时失调，表现为肺的宣降失司。肺失宣降的病机变化主要有气机失调，津液不布和气血郁滞三大类。

3.1 Qì Dynamic Disorders

3.1.1 Lung Qì Depression

The lung governs qì. When upward, downward, inward, and outward movement are orderly, the qì dynamic of the entire body is coordinated and harmonious. Obstruction by evil qì or the retention of pathologic substances can prevent lung qì from performing upward diffusion to the upper and outer body, and depurative downbearing to the lower and inner body. When upbearing and downbearing break down, the qì dynamic is most likely to stagnate in the chest, which leads to lung qì congestion. This manifests in such symptoms as oppression and constraint in the chest, a sensation like obstruction in the chest and diaphragm, and distention and pain in the chest and back. The "Great Treatise on the Essentials of Supreme Truth" in the *Sù Wèn* ("Plain Questions") states: "All types of huffing and depression of qì belong to the lung." This is a concise summary of this pathomechanism of lung qì depression block. *zhǐ qiào* (*ké*) (Aurantii Fructus) and *jié gěng* (Platycodonis Radix) are most commonly used to treat this condition, since one upbears and the other downbears, with the effect that they together diffuse lung block. In cases of concurrent phlegm obstruction, *èr chén tāng* (Two Matured Ingredients Decoction) is used.

In addition, affect-mind dissatisfaction can also lead to lung qì depression. As explained in the chapter, "Depression" in the *Yī Biǎn* ("Lancing Stones of Medicine"):

> "This refers to a failure of clear qì to ascend and of turbid qì to descend. In that case, clear and turbid all exit into the lung, causing greater yīn to lose its regulatory power. Vital qì fails to rise, and absorbed qì fails to descend. Upper body and lower body do not interact and depression arises."

In the chapter, "Depression" in the *Lín Zhèng Zhǐ Nán Yī Àn* ("A Clinical Guide with Case Histories"), Yè Tiān-Shì used the method of "opening and downbearing lung qì" to treat depression patterns. This treatment principle is formulated on precisely this notion of a breakdown in lung diffusion and downbearing. When a binding depression of phlegm and qì arises in the throat, this is caused by liver depression with qì stagnation and by phlegm and qì obstructing the lung and ascending counterflow into the throat. It is treated appropriately by moving qì and opening depression, and by downbearing qì and transforming phlegm. The recommended formula is *bàn xià hòu pò tāng* (Pinellia and Officinal Magnolia Bark Decoction) from the *Jīn Guì Yào Lüè* ("Essential Prescriptions of the Golden Coffer").

Bàn Xià Tāng 半夏厚朴汤 (Pinellia and Officinal Magnolia Bark Decoction)
bàn xià 半夏 (Pinelliae Rhizoma, pinellia) *zǐ sū zǐ* 紫苏子 (Perillae Fructus, perilla fruit) *hòu pò* 厚朴 (Magnoliae Officinalis Cortex, officinal magnolia bark) *fú líng* 茯苓 (Poria, poria) *shēng jiāng* 生姜 (Zingiberis Rhizoma Recens, fresh ginger)

气机失调

肺气郁滞

肺主气, 升降出入有序, 则全身气机协调. 邪气阻滞或病理产物停留, 肺气不能向上向外升宣, 亦不能向下向内肃降, 升降失司, 气机最易停滞在胸中, 导致肺气壅塞, 表现为胸闷不舒、胸膈似阻、胸背胀痛等症. 《素问•至真要大论》: "诸气膹郁, 皆属于肺" 正是对肺气闭郁这一病机的高度概括. 最常用枳壳、桔梗, 一升一降以宣通肺闭. 若兼痰阻, 则用枳桔二陈汤.

此外，情志不遂亦可导致肺气郁滞。如《医述•郁》说："所谓者，清气不升，浊气不降也。然清浊升降皆出于肺，使太阴失治节之权，不唯生气不升，收气亦不降，上下不交而郁成也。" 叶天士《临证指南医案•郁》中用"开降肺气"治疗郁证，就是根据肺的宣降失职而制定的法则。如痰气郁结咽喉，就是肝郁气滞，痰气阻肺，上逆咽喉而成。治宜行气开郁，降气化痰。方选《金匮要略》半夏厚朴汤（半夏、紫苏、厚朴、茯苓、生姜）。

3.1.2 Counterflow Ascent of Lung Qì

When the lung's diffusion and downbearing are impaired, lung qì becomes blocked. When this progresses further, lung qì fails to bear downward and instead ascends counterflow. This is the pathomechanism of counterflow ascent of lung qì. This manifests in the symptoms of cough, hasty panting, dyspnea, and phlegm-drool congestion. Depending on differences in the disease cause, symptoms manifest in particular ways:

A. Evil Heat Invading the Lung

When evil heat invades the lung and steams therein, or when it boils fluids down to phlegm so that phlegm-heat blazes intensely inside the lung, this distresses lung qì and forces it to ascend counterflow. The resulting patterns of repletion heat in the lung manifest in cough, panting, and rough breathing, high voice and gushing breath, coughing and spitting of turbid malodorous yellow phlegm, a thick and slimy yellow tongue fur, and a slippery and rapid pulse.

This is explained in the "Treatise on Needling Heat" in the *Sù Wèn* ("Plain Questions"): "Lung heat disease manifests first in sudden shivering reversal with raised body hair, aversion to wind and cold, yellow tongue fur, and generalized heat effusion. Struggling heat then causes cough and panting, wandering pain in the anterior chest and back, inability to sigh deeply, and unbearable headache." Struggling heat resulting in cough and panting refers directly to the pathomechanism of lung qì and evil heat contending with each other and causing lung qì block and counterflow ascent of lung qì. The chapter, "Lung Repletion Heat" in the *Qiān Jīn Yào Fāng* ("A Thousand Gold Pieces Prescriptions") also explains:

> "When a patient suffers from distention of the lung, discharge of sweat like dewdrops, qì ascent and panting counterflow, congestion in the throat, and an appearance as if about to retch, this is called lung repletion heat."

This quotation also points out that an excessive exuberance of evil heat in the lung can lead to counterflow ascent of lung qì.

This condition is treated by clearing heat and draining the lung, and by downbearing qì and calming panting. The appropriate formula is *má xìng shí gān tāng* (Ephedra, Apricot Kernel, Gypsum, and Licorice Decoction) from the *Shāng Hán Lùn* ("On Cold Damage") in combination with *wěi jīng tāng* (Phragmites Stem Decoction) from the *Qiān Jīn Yào Fāng* ("A Thousand Gold Pieces Prescriptions").

Má Xìng Shí Gān Tāng 麻杏石甘汤 (Ephedra, Apricot Kernel, Gypsum, and Licorice Decoction) with *Wěi Jīng Tāng* 苇茎汤 (Phragmites Stem Decoction)
má huáng 麻黄 (Ephedrae Herba, ephedra)
xìng rén 杏仁 (Armeniacae Semen, apricot kernel)
shí gāo 石膏 (Gypsum Fibrosum, gypsum)
gān cǎo 甘草 (Glycyrrhizae Radix, licorice root)
Plus:
táo rén 桃仁 (Persicae Semen, peach kernel)
dōng guā zǐ 冬瓜子 (Benincasae Semen, wax gourd seed)
yì yǐ rén 薏苡仁 (Coicis Semen, coix)
wěi jīng 芦茎 (Phragmititis Caulis, phragmites stem)

B. Cold Evil Invading the Lung

When cold evil invades the lung and disturbs diffusion and downbearing, cold phlegm congeals and stagnates, congests lung qì, and causes it to ascend counterflow. This leads to patterns of cold repletion in the lung, which manifest in cough, panting, and wheezing, oppression in the chest and tightness of qì, a profusion of clear white thin phlegm, a slippery white tongue fur, and a tight stringlike pulse.

The chapter, "Forms of Disease from Evil Qì in the Viscera and Bowels" in the *Líng Shū* ("The Magic Pivot") explains: "A cold body and drinking cold fluids damages the lung. These two kinds of cold affect each other, damaging both the center and the outside. This causes qì to counterflow and move upward." The chapter, "Cold in the Lung" in the *Shèng Jì Zǒng Lù* ("Sages' Salvation Records") states: "If the body is struck by cold evil, the result is cough and nasal congestion, spittle and turbid snivel, a hoarse broken voice, and aversion to cold as after a soaking." This describes how cold, being a yīn evil, can block the interstices of the flesh and impede lung qì. By congealing liquid and forming phlegm, this leads to lung congestion and qì counterflow.

This condition is treated by resolving the exterior with warmth and acridity, and by diffusing the lung and calming panting. The appropriate formula is *má huáng tāng* (Ephedra Decoction) from the *Shāng Hán Lùn* ("On Cold Damage") with the addition of *bàn xià* (Pinelliae Rhizoma), *fú líng* (Poria), and *zǐ sū zǐ* (Perillae Fructus).

Má Huáng Tāng 麻黄汤 (Ephedra Decoction)
má huáng 麻黄 (Ephedrae Herba, ephedra)
guì zhī 桂枝 (Cinnamomi Ramulus, cinnamon twig)
xìng rén 杏仁 (Armeniacae Semen, apricot kernel)
gān cǎo 甘草 (Glycyrrhizae Radix, licorice)
Plus:
bàn xià 半夏 (Pinelliae Rhizoma, pinellia)
fú líng 茯苓 (Poria, poria)
zǐ sū zǐ 紫苏子 (Perillae Fructus, perilla fruit)

C. Dryness Evil Invading the Lung

When dryness evil invades the lung, it astringes lung qì. As a result it can inhibit lung qì, disturb diffusion and downbearing, and cause counterflow ascent of lung qì. This manifests in cough, panting, and dry mouth, and in dry cough with scant phlegm that is not easily expectorated.

The chapter, "Differentiating Cough by the Six Qì and not Restricting it to an Account of Cold" in the *Rú Mén Shì Qīn* ("Confucian Filiality") states:

> "When dryness overwhelms the lung, it manifests in qì congestion and inhibition, pain inside the hundred joints, sweating head and face, alternating heat effusion and aversion to cold, desiccated skin, delicate dry itchy sores, constipated and rough defecation, and thick sticky sniffle and spittle."

The "Section on Phlegm" in the *Yī Xué Rù Mén* ("The Gateway to Medicine") also states:

> "When [dryness phlegm] ascends into the lung, it manifests in increasingly parched body hair, a face that is white as dry bones, and in dryness of the mouth and throat, cough, and hasty panting. Being called 'dryness phlegm,' this type of phlegm is astringed and difficult to expel."

These two quotations illustrate the pathomechanism by which dryness evil invading the lung by way of congesting lung qì causes cough with counterflow qì ascent and ungratifying expectoration of phlegm.

This condition is treated by clearing the lung and moistening dryness, amd by downbearing qì and transforming phlegm. The recommended formula is *sāng xìng tāng* (Mulberry Leaf and Apricot Kernel Decoction) from the *Wēn Bìng Tiáo Bian* ("Systematized Identification of Warm Diseases") with the addition of *jié gěng* (Platycodonis Radix), *qián hú* (Peucedani Radix), *mài mén dōng* (Ophiopogonis Radix), and *zhī mǔ* (Anemarrhenae Rhizoma).

Sāng Xìng Tāng 桑杏汤 (Mulberry Leaf and Apricot Kernel Decoction)
sāng yè 桑叶 (Mori Folium, mulberry leaf)
xìng rén 杏仁 (Armeniacae Semen, apricot kernel
shā shēn 沙参 (Adenophorae seu Glehniae Radix, adenophora/glehnia
bèi mǔ 贝母 (Fritillariae Bulbus, fritillaria)
dàn dòu chǐ 淡豆豉 (Sojae Semen Praeparatum, fermented soybean)
qín pí 秦皮 (Fraxini Cortex, ash)
lí pí 梨皮 (Pyri Exocarpium, pear peel)
Plus:
jié gěng 桔梗 (Platycodonis Radix, platycodon)
qián hú 前胡 (Peucedani Radix, peucedanum)
mài mén dōng 麦门冬 (Ophiopogonis Radix, ophiopogon)
zhī mǔ 知母 (Anemarrhenae Rhizoma, anemarrhena)

Alternatively, *bèi mǔ guā lóu sǎn* (Fritillaria and Trichosanthes Powder) from the *Yī Xué Xīn Wù* ("Medical Insights") with modifications is used.

Bèi Mǔ Sǎn 贝母栝蒌散 (Fritillaria and Trichosanthes Powder)
bèi mǔ 贝母 (Fritillariae Bulbus, fritillaria)
guā lóu pí 栝楼皮 (Trichosanthis Pericarpium, trichosanthes rind)
tiān huā fěn 天花粉 (Trichosanthis Radix, trichosanthes root)
fú líng 茯苓 (Poria, poria)
jú hóng 橘红 (Citri Reticulatae Pericarpium Rubrum, red tangerine peel)
jié gěng 桔梗 (Platycodonis Radix, platycodon)

D. Summerheat Evil Invading the Lung

When summerheat evil invades the lung, its torrid steamy heat disturbs diffusion and downbearing and causes lung qì to ascend counterflow, leading to summerheat cough. It manifests in dizzy head, heat effusion, aversion to cold, thirst, heavy cumbersome head and body, cough with scant phlegm that is not easily expectorated, yellow urine, and a red tongue with a thin yellow tongue fur.

The chapter, "Cough" in the *Lèi Zhèng Zhì Cái* ("Systematized Patterns with Clear-Cut Treatments") states:

> "Summerheat cough means that the steaming of summerheat-heat produces cough, while summerheat-wind assails lung defense. The inch pulse is large, the throat itchy, and the mouth thirsty… When summerheat concurs with dampness, the result is cough with thick phlegm, qì obstruction, and inhibited urination."

This illustrates how summerheat-heat or summerheat-damp invading the lung makes lung qì ascend counterflow, which can lead to cough.

This condition is treated by clearing heat and flushing summerheat, and by downbearing qì and suppressing cough. The recommended formula is *qīng liáng dí shǔ tāng* (Cool Clearing Summerheat-Flushing Decoction) from the *Shí Bìng Lùn* ("On Seasonal Diseases") with the addition of *xìng rén* (Armeniacae Semen) and *guā lóu pí* (Trichosanthis Pericarpium).

Qīng Liáng Dí Shǔ Tāng 清凉涤暑法 (Cool Clearing Summerheat-Flushing Decoction)
bái biăn dòu 白扁豆 (Lablab Semen Album, lablab)
qīng hāo 青蒿 (Artemisiae Annuae Herba, sweet wormwood)
lián qiào 连翘 (Forsythiae Fructus, forsythia)
fú líng 茯苓 (Poria, poria)
huá shí 滑石 (Talcum, talcum)
tōng căo 通草 (Tetrapanacis Medulla, rice-paper plant pith)
gān căo 甘草 (Glycyrrhizae Radix, licorice)
Plus:
xìng rén 杏仁(Armeniacae Semen, apricot kernel)
guā lóu pí 栝楼皮(Trichosanthis Pericarpium, trichosanthes rind)

肺气上逆

肺失宣降，肺气闭塞，进一步发展，肺气不降，反而上逆，可形成肺气上逆的病机，表现为咳嗽、喘促、呼吸困难、痰涎壅盛诸症。并随致病原因不同，症状表现各异:

邪热犯肺，热邪熏蒸，或热邪煎熬，炼液为痰，肺中痰热炽盛，逼迫肺气上逆，而致肺的实热证，表现为咳喘气粗、声高息涌、咳吐黄浊臭痰，舌苔黄而厚腻，脉象滑数等症。如《素问•刺热论》说:"肺热病者，先淅然厥起毫毛，恶风寒，舌上黄，身热。热争则咳喘，痛走膺背，不得太息，头痛不堪。”热争则咳喘，即言肺气与邪热相互搏击，肺气闭塞，肺气上逆的病机。《千金要方•肺实热》也说：“病苦肺胀，汗出若露，上气喘逆，咽中塞，如欲呕状，名曰肺实热也。”均指出肺中邪热太盛，可致肺气上逆。治宜清热泻肺，降气平喘。方选《伤寒论》麻杏石甘汤（麻黄、杏仁、石膏、甘草）合《千金要方》苇茎汤（桃仁、冬瓜仁、薏苡仁、苇茎）。

寒邪犯肺，宣降失司，寒痰凝滞，肺气壅塞，肺气上逆，可致肺的寒实证，表现为咳喘哮鸣、胸闷气紧、痰多色白清稀，舌苔白滑，脉弦紧。如《灵枢•邪气脏腑病形篇》说：“形寒饮冷则伤肺，以其两寒相感，中外皆伤，故气逆而上行。”《圣济总录•肺中寒》云：“苟为寒邪所中，则有咳而鼻塞，唾浊涕，语声嘶破，洒淅恶寒之证。”阐述寒为阴邪，闭塞肌腠，阻碍肺气，凝津成痰，而致肺塞气逆。治宜辛温解表，宣肺平喘。方选《伤寒论》麻黄汤加半夏、茯苓、苏子。

燥邪犯肺，枯涩肺气，可致肺气不利，宣降失司，肺气上逆。表现为咳喘口燥，干咳痰少，不易咯出等症。如《儒门事亲•嗽分六气毋拘以寒述》云：“燥乘肺者，气壅不利，百节内痛，头面汗出，寒热往来，皮肤干枯，细疮燥痒，大便秘涩，涕唾稠粘。”《医学入门•痰门》也云：“升于肺，多毛焦面白如枯骨，咽干口燥、咳嗽、喘促、名曰燥痰，其痰涩而难出。”两条阐明了燥邪犯肺，通过滞塞肺气，而致咳逆上气，咯痰不爽的病机。治宜清肺润燥，降气化痰。方选《温病条辨》桑杏汤（桑叶、杏仁、沙参、象贝母、淡豆豉、栀皮、梨皮）加桔梗、前胡、麦冬、知母。

或用《医学心悟》贝母瓜蒌散（贝母、瓜蒌壳、花粉、茯苓、橘红、桔梗）加减。

暑邪犯肺，暑热炎蒸，宣降失常，肺气上逆，可致暑咳。表现为头晕、发热、恶寒、口渴、头身困重、咳嗽痰少，不易咯出，尿黄、舌红苔薄黄等症。如《类证治裁•咳嗽》云：“暑嗽，暑热蒸嗽，及暑风袭入肺卫，寸脉大，喉痒口渴。…暑兼湿，咳而痰稠，气阻溺涩。”说明暑热或暑湿犯肺，肺气上逆，可引起咳嗽。治宜清热涤暑，降气止咳。用《时病论》清凉涤暑法（滑石、生甘草、青蒿、白扁豆、连翘、白茯苓、通草）加杏仁、瓜蒌壳。

Literature Review of Qì Dynamic Disorders

🕮 *Jīn Guì Yào Lüè* ("Essential Prescriptions of the Golden Coffer"), "Pulse Symptoms and Treatments of Lung Wilting, Lung Welling-Abscess, Cough, and Qì Ascent"

> "When there is heat in the upper burner, cough causes lung wilting."

This quotation points out how heat in the upper burner scorches the lung and distresses lung qì, forcing it to ascend counterflow. When the resulting cough is chronic, it damages the lung, forming lung wilting.

🕮 *Pǔ Jì Fāng* ("Universal Salvation Formulary"), "Cough"

> "The lung governs qì, and qì is yáng. When yáng is exuberant, it engenders heat. This always results in disorder in the viscera and bowels, rough inhibited flow in the channels and network vessels, evil heat restraining the upper burner, inhibition of the qì dynamic, accumulations and gatherings due to phlegm repletion, and vexation and fullness in the chest. This causes cough."

This quotation illustrates how an excessive exuberance of yáng heat in the lung causes phlegm-heat blocking the lung, and counterflow ascent of lung qì. This leads to the pathomechanical changes of cough, vexation, and fullness.

🕮 *Yī Lín Shéng Mò* ("Level Line Ink of the Forest of Medicine"), "Cough"

> "In cases of heat phlegm, phlegm stirs because of fire. Perhaps a liking for roasted foods, for liquor and foods containing yeast, or for fatty, rich, oily and slimy foods has caused them to accumulate inside the body and transform into thick phlegm. This causes disease and manifests in fullness of the chest, rapid breathing, and phlegm panting and inhibition."

This quotation describes the pathomechanism by which phlegm-heat amassing and congesting lung qì causes counterflow ascent of lung qì, which results in panting and cough.

🕮 *Dú Yī Suí Bǐ* ("Informal Essays on Reading Medical Texts"), "Treatise on Cough"

> "Sudden cough with continuous sound that cannot be stopped even temporarily means that cold and wind have followed the breath and assailed the lung. In this case, wind assailing the lung has caused cough…External contraction of wind-cold with aversion to cold and heat effusion also mostly manifests with cough. This is because wind-cold enters the lung from the channels. It should be treated first in the exterior

> by dissipating, and in enduring cases, also by clearing and downbearing. The sound of the cough is clear and loud, and identical during the day and night."

This quotation describes the pathomechanism by which wind-cold assailing the lung causes impaired diffusion and downbearing of the lung, counterflow ascent of lung qì, and incessant cough.

📖 *Bǐ Huā Yī Jìng* ("Bǐ-Huā's Medical Mirror"), "Lung Section"

> "Lung cold patterns are mostly due to external contraction. The right inch pulse will invariably be slow, and the symptoms are clear snivel, cough, aversion to cold, and a withered white facial complexion. The clear snivel indicates that cold is contending with humor...The cough indicates that metal is afraid of the cold....The aversion to cold indicates that yīn is avoiding its own kind."

This quotation points out that wind-cold invading the lung and impairing its ability to diffuse and downbear can lead to the symptoms of cough, clear snivel, and aversion to cold. Furthermore, it also expounds the pathomechanism that causes these manifestations.

📖 *Lín Zhèng Zhǐ Nán Yī Àn* ("A Clinical Guide with Case Histories"), "Wheezing," Xú's case history

> "When cold evil invades the back transport points, which internally are connected to the lung tie, abiding evil can obstruct qì and phlegm. This manifests in the symptoms of panting and inability to sleep."

The same text points out in the commentary on the patterns of "Panting":

> "In most cases of repletion with resulting cold, the condition is invariably complicated by congealed phlegm and abiding rheum, which interfere in the upper body and obstruct qì."

This quotation describes the pathomechanism by which cold phlegm congealing in the lung and counterflow ascent of lung qì lead to panting counterflow.

📖 *Zhèng Zhì Huì Bǔ* ("Combined Supplements to Patterns and Treatment"), "Wheezing Disease"

> "Internally, there can be congested qì; externally, there can be an untimely contraction; in the diaphragm, there can be stubbornly adhering phlegm. When these three unite with each other, they can block the airways. Their contending and attacking produces sound, which manifests in the symptom of wheezing."

This quotation describes the pathomechanism by which enduring phlegm panting causes phlegm turbidity obstructing the lung and counterflow ascent of lung qì, which leads to wheezing.

📖 *Zhèng Yīn Mài Zhì* ("Pathoconditions: Causes, Pulses, and Treatments"), "Dryness Damage Cough"

> "Climatic changes in the sky cause dryness and fissures. Dryness is formed out of fire, and the lung is damaged by dryness... [The symptoms are] thirst and generalized heat effusion, redness and inhibited voiding of stool and urine, qì counterflow panting and cough, red face and parched lips, and dry cough without phlegm."

This quotation describes how dryness evil damaging the lung can lead to counterflow ascent of lung qì, resulting in such manifestations as dry cough and qì counterflow.

📖 *Lèi Zhèng Zhì Cái* ("Systematized Patterns with Clear-Cut Treatments"), "Symptom of Dryness"

> "When dryness is located in the upper body, it invariably overwhelms the lung, causing dryness cough. Fire inside the lung manifests in dry cough."

This quotation describes the pathomechanism by which dryness evil overwhelming the lung and the resulting counterflow ascent of lung qì can lead to dry cough.

📖 *Zhèng Yīn Mài Zhì* ("Pathoconditions: Causes, Pulses, and Treatments"), "Cough"

> "The signs of summerheat damage cough are generalized heat effusion with taking of fluids; internal heat and vexing dryness, but external aversion to cold; possible generalized pain and thirst; and cough with bodily fatigue. These are the signs of summerheat damaging lung qì. Regarding the cause of summerheat damage cough, it happens in the summer or fall. Perhaps a person with qì vacuity and generalized heat encountered encroachment by summerheat dampness. Or a person with severe heat in the center happened to contract a seasonal condition. Internal and external [conditions] attack each other, brew in the region of the chest and stomach, and suffocate the lung. This results in summerheat-damp cough."

This quotation describes the manifestations of summerheat cough due to summerheat-heat damaging the lung and counterflow ascent of lung qì. In addition, it analyzes the pathomechanism of summerheat-heat suffocating the lung with counterflow ascent of lung qì.

📖 *Yī Mén Fǎ Lǜ* ("Axioms of Medicine"), "Section on Cough"

> "In diseases governed by the six qì, wind, fire, heat, dampness, dryness, and cold can all overwhelm the lung and lead to cough. Among these, dampness cough is really an aspect associated with the other five qì of wind, fire, heat, dryness, or cold.

> Cough that results from wind overcoming the lung manifests in sweating, headache, and in inhibition of phlegm-drool. Cough that results from fire overcoming the lung manifests in rapid panting with congestion and counterflow, and in sniffle and spittle that contain blood.
>
> Cough that results from heat overcoming the lung manifests in rapid panting; redness and tidal heat in the face; in severe cases of heat exuberance in the center, in paradoxical cold in the four extremities; and when the heat shifts into the lower body, in intolerable diarrhea. Cough that results from dryness overcoming the lung manifests in dry skin and body hair, delicate sores that are damp and itch, and in constipation from adhering phlegm.
>
> Cough that results from cold overcoming the lung manifests in aversion to cold without sweating, nasal congestion and generalized pain, heat effusion, and agitated vexation. When internal stirring of damp phlegm causes cough, even though the complicating factors (wind, fire, heat, dryness, or cold) are not identical, once it overwhelms the lung, the result is the same."

This quotation describes comprehensively how an external contraction of the six excesses causes lung qì block, breakdown of diffusion and downbearing, and counterflow ascent of lung qì, which manifests clinically in different types of cough.

文献综述

《金匮要略•肺痿肺痈咳嗽上气病脉证治》曰: "热在上焦者，因咳为肺痿。" 指出热在上焦，熏灼于肺，逼迫肺气上逆为咳，咳久伤肺则成肺痿。

《普济方•咳嗽》曰: "肺主于气，气为阳，阳盛则生热也，皆脏腑不调，经络痞涩，邪热克于上焦，气道不利，痰实积聚，胸中烦满，故令咳嗽也。" 阐明肺中阳热过盛，痰热闭肺，肺气上逆，引起咳嗽烦满的病机变化。

《医林绳墨•咳嗽》曰: "热痰者，痰因火动，或好食炙煿、酒曲、膏梁、油腻等物，蓄积于内，化为稠痰，故发而为胸满气急，痰喘不利。" 论述痰热蓄积，壅塞肺气，肺气上逆而喘咳的病机。

《读医随笔•论咳嗽》曰: "卒然咳嗽，连声不可暂止者，此冷风随呼吸而袭肺也。此风袭肺则咳嗽。…外感风寒，恶寒发热，亦多有咳嗽者。此风寒由经入肺也，宜先表散，久则兼清降。其咳声清响，而昼夜相等。" 论述风寒袭肺，肺失宣降，肺气上逆，咳嗽连声不止的病机。

《笔花医镜•肺部》曰:“肺寒之证，外感居多，脉右寸必迟，其症为清涕，为咳嗽，为恶寒，为面色痿白。清涕者，寒搏其液也。…咳嗽者，金畏其寒也。…恶寒者，阴忌其类也。”不仅阐述寒邪犯肺，肺失宣降引起咳嗽、清涕、恶寒的症状，而且进一步阐述了引起这些表现的病机。

《临证指南医案•哮》徐案曰:“寒邪入背俞，内合于肺系，宿邪阻气阻痰，病发喘不得卧。”又在《喘》证的按语中指出“大凡实而寒者，必挟凝痰宿饮，上干阻气。”阐述了寒痰凝肺，肺气上逆，引起喘逆的病机。

《证治汇补•哮病》曰:“内有壅塞之气，外有非时之感，膈有胶固之痰，三者相合，闭拒气道，搏击有声。发为哮证。”论述痰喘日久，痰浊阻肺，肺气上逆可引起哮证的病机。

《症因脉治•伤燥咳嗽》中指出病因为“天行燥裂，燥从火化，肺被燥伤。”症状为“口渴身热，二便赤涩，喘咳气逆，面赤唇焦，干咳无痰。”论述燥邪伤肺，可致肺气上逆，而引起干咳气逆等诸多表现。

《类证治裁•燥症》曰:“燥在上，必乘肺，为燥咳。肺中有火为干咳。”论述燥邪乘肺，肺气上逆，可致干咳的病机。

《症因脉治•咳嗽》曰:“伤暑咳嗽之症，身热引饮，内热烦燥，外反恶寒，或身痛口渴，咳嗽身倦，此暑伤肺气之症也。伤暑咳嗽之因，时值夏秋，或气虚身热，触冒暑湿；或热甚于中，偶感时行，内外夹攻，蒸酿胸胃之间，上熏于肺，则暑湿咳嗽作矣。”不仅论述暑热伤肺，肺气上逆所致暑咳的表现，而且深刻分析暑热熏肺，引起肺气上逆的病机。

《医门法律•咳嗽门》曰:“六气主病，风、火、热、湿、燥、寒皆能乘肺，皆足以致咳。其湿咳即分属于风、火、热、燥、寒五气之中也。风乘肺咳，汗出头痛，痰涎不利。火乘肺咳，喘急壅逆，涕唾见血。热乘肺咳，喘急，面赤潮热，甚者热盛于中，四末反寒，热移于下，便泄无度。燥乘肺咳，皮毛干槁，细疮湿痒，痰胶便秘。寒乘于肺，恶寒无汗，鼻塞身疼，发热躁烦。至于湿痰内动为咳，又必因风，因火，因热，因燥，因寒，所挟不相同，至乘肺则一也。”全面论述外感六淫，肺气闭塞，宣降失职，肺气上逆所致各种咳嗽的临床表现。

Summary of Lung Qì Disorders
1. Lung Qì Depression Oppression and constraint in the chest, a sensation like obstruction in the chest and diaphragm, distention and pain in the chest and back. 2. Counterflow Ascent of Lung Qì *Phlegm-heat congesting the lung*: Cough, panting, and rough breathing; high voice and gushing breath; coughing and spitting of turbid malodorous yellow phlegm. *Cold phlegm congealing in the lung*: Cough, panting, and wheezing; oppression in the chest and tightness of qì; copious clear-white thin phlegm. *Dryness evil invading the lung*: Cough, panting, and dry mouth; dry cough with scant phlegm that is not easily expectorated. *Summerheat-heat assailing the lung*: Dizzy head, heat effusion, heavy cumbersome head and body, cough with scant phlegm that is difficult to expel.

肺气失调
肺气郁滞 胸闷不舒，胸膈似阻，胸背胀痛。 肺气上逆 痰热壅肺—咳喘气粗，声高息涌，咳吐黄浊臭痰。 寒痰凝肺—咳喘哮鸣，胸闷气紧，痰多色白清稀。 燥邪犯肺—咳喘口燥，干咳痰少，不易咯出。 暑热袭肺—头晕，发热，头身困重，咳嗽痰少难出。

3.2 Non-Distribution of the Fluids

The lung governs regulation of the waterways and is the upper source of water. Through the diffusion and depurative downbearing of lung qì, the fluids, with the triple burner as the thoroughfare, are distributed throughout the entire body and provide for the necessary vital activities in the human body. Any number of causes can influence the lung's ability to diffuse and downbear. When the lung fails to diffuse, it can lead to obstructions in the distribution of fluids and sweat, and to a failure to dissipate water qì to the outside. When the lung fails to depurate and downbear, waste water cannot be moved down into the bladder, turned into urine, and discharged from the body. It causes it to collect in the lung and transform into phlegm, rheum, dampness, and water, resulting in a variety of pathomechanical changes.

津液不布

肺主通调水道，为水之上源。肺气宣发肃降，水液以三焦为通道，敷布全身，供给人体生命活动的需要。各种原因影响肺的宣降功能，肺失宣发，可使津液和汗液输布受阻，水气不得外散；肺失肃降，废水不能下输膀胱，变成尿液排出体外，停滞于肺，转化为痰、饮、湿、水,引起多种病机变化。

3.2.1 Internal Collection of Water Qì

When lung qì is blocked and depressed, diffusion and downbearing break down, and the fluids collect instead of being distributed by the upper burner. Spilling into the skin, this manifests as water swelling, indicating the upflow of water to its higher source. It is characterized by a rapid onset and mostly manifests in severe swelling in the head and face and upper half of the body, as well as short voidings of scant urine.

The chapter "Understanding Sickness by Examination of the Cubit Skin" in the *Líng Shū* ("The Magic Pivot") states:

> "One sees slight swelling of the eye nest, as [in one] newly arisen from sleep; the neck pulse stirs, and there is frequent cough. When you press the hands and feet, they pit but do not spring back. [All this constitutes] wind water skin distention."

Wind water is closely related to the pathomechanism of breakdown of the lung's diffusion and downbearing with water qì flooding.

The commentary to the "Treatise on Points for Water and Heat" in the *Sù Wèn* ("Elementary Questions") states:

> "In sweating that is related to [excessive] taxation from display of valor, the mysterious mansions [i.e. sweat pores] are open; in sweating with exposure to wind, the mysterious mansions are closed. If the mysterious mansions are closed, sweat cannot be discharged. Instead, it stays hidden under the skin and transforms into water. Because the water is a result of wind, it is called wind water."

In the context of discussing *mài mén dōng yǐn zǐ* (Ophiopogon Drink), Kitayama Tomomatsuko, author of *Yī Fāng Kǎo Shéng Qiān* ("Corrections to 'Medical Remedies Researched'"), in the chapter, "Water Swelling," states:

> "When the lung is hot, it loses its command over downbearing. It becomes unable to regulate the waterways and transport water downward into the bladder. Instead, water soaks into the upper source, oozes into the skin, and causes water swelling. Physicians rarely understand this."

These quotations all describe the pathomechanism by which impaired diffusion and downbearing of the lung and non-distribution of fluids can form water swelling.

On the basis of differences in the nature of the external evil, when wind-cold blocks the lung, *má huáng jiā zhú tāng* (Ephedra Decoction Plus White Atractylodes) from the *Shāng Hán Lùn* ("On Cold Damage") is used *má huáng tāng* (Ephedra Decoction) with *bái zhú* (Atractylodis Macrocephalae Rhizoma) added.

Má Huáng Jiā Zhú Tāng 麻黄加朮汤
(Ephedra Decoction Plus White Atractylodes)

má huáng 麻黄 (Ephedrae Herba, ephedra)
guì zhī 桂枝 (Cinnamomi Ramulus, cinnamon twig)
xìng rén(杏仁 (Armeniacae Semen, apricot kernel)
gān cǎo 甘草 (Glycyrrhizae Radix, licorice)
with:
bái zhú 白朮 (Atractylodis Macrocephalae Rhizoma, white atractylodes)

For wind-heat invading the lung, *yuè bì jiā zhú tāng* (Spleen-Effusing Decoction Plus White Atractylodes) from the *Shāng Hán Lùn* ("On Cold Damage") is used.

Yuè Bì Jiā Zhú Tāng 越婢加朮汤
(Spleen-Effusing Decoction Plus White Atractylodes)

má huáng 麻黄 (Ephedrae Herba, ephedra)
shí gāo 石膏 (Gypsum Fibrosum, gypsum)
shēng jiāng 生姜 (Zingiberis Rhizoma Recens, fresh ginger)
gān cǎo 甘草 (Glycyrrhizae Radix, licorice)
bái zhú 白朮 (Atractylodis Macrocephalae Rhizoma, white atractylodes)
dà zǎo 大枣 (Jujubae Fructus, jujube)

And for damp-heat invading the lung, *má huáng lián qiào chì xiǎo dòu tāng* (Ephedra, Forsythia, and Rice Bean Decoction) from the *Shāng Hán Lùn* ("On Cold Damage") is used.

Má Huáng Lián Qiào Chì Xiǎo Dòu Tāng 麻黄连翘赤小豆汤
(Ephedra, Forsythia, and Rice Bean Decoction)

má huáng 麻黄 (Ephedrae Herba, ephedra)
lián qiào 连翘 (Forsythiae Fructus, forsythia)
chì xiǎo dòu 赤小豆 (Phaseoli Semen, rice bean)
bái pí 白皮 (Catalpae Cortex, catalpae bark)
xìng rén 杏仁 (Armeniacae Semen, apricot kernel)
shēng jiāng 生姜 (Zingiberis Rhizoma Recens, fresh ginger)
dà zǎo 大枣 (Jujubae Fructus, jujube)
gān cǎo 甘草 (Glycyrrhizae Radix, licorice)

水气内停

肺气闭郁, 宣降失职, 津液停聚, 上焦不布, 泛溢肌肤, 发为水肿. 此为水泛高原, 发病急, 多见头面、上半身肿甚, 小便短少. 如《灵枢•论疾诊尺》云: "视人之目巢上微痈, 如新卧起状, 其颈脉动, 时咳, 按其手足上, 窅而不起者, 风水肤胀也. " 风水与肺失宣降, 水气泛滥的病机有密切关系. 正如《黄帝内经素问》对水热穴论注曰: "劳勇汗出则玄府开, 汗出逢风则玄府闭, 玄府闭已则余汗未出, 内伏皮肤, 传化为水, 从风而水, 故名风水. " 北山友松子《医方考绳愆•水肿•麦门冬饮》云: "肺热则失其下降之令, 不能通调水道, 下输膀胱, 渍于高原, 淫于皮肤则作水肿, 医罕明乎此, 实土导水皆不能愈. " 均深刻阐述了肺失宣降, 津液失布形成水肿的病机. 根据外邪性质的差异, 风寒闭肺, 用《伤寒论》麻黄加术汤（麻黄汤加白术）; 风热犯肺, 用《伤寒论》越婢加术汤; 湿热犯肺, 用《伤寒论》麻黄连翘赤小豆汤（麻黄、连翘、赤小豆、梓白皮、杏仁、生姜、大枣、甘草）。

3.2.2 Damp Turbidity Flooding Upward

When the lung's diffusion and downbearing are impaired, the fluids do not move, but instead transform into dampness. They collect in the upper burner where they often combine with heat. This forms a pattern of upper burner damp-heat. It can manifest in symptoms like aversion to cold and heat effusion, cough with white phlegm, unsurfaced generalized heat, heavy and aching head and body, oppression in the chest and glomus in the stomach duct, and a thick slimy pale yellow tongue fur.

The chapter, "Damp-Heat Disease" in the *Wēn Bìng Zōng Héng* ("Warm Disease: A Comprehensive Review") explains:

> "Upper burner damp-heat patterns … mean that the evil qì of damp-heat has entered through the mouth or nose and assailed the lung. This leads to such conditions as disturbed diffusion and downbearing of lung qì, abnormalities in the external defense function, and malfunctions in the fluid metabolism."

This condition is treated by clearing heat and transforming dampness, and by diffusing the lung and eliminating phlegm. The recommended formula is *sān rén tāng* (Three Kernels Decoction) from the *Wēn Bìng Tiáo Bian* ("Systematized Identification of Warm Diseases") with the addition of *zǐ wǎn* (Asteris Radix) and *pí pá yè* (Eriobotryae Folium).

Sān Rén Tāng 三仁汤 (Three Kernels Decoction)
xìng rén 杏仁 (Armeniacae Semen, apricot kernel)
bái kòu rén 砂仁 (Amomi Fructus Rotundus, cardamom)

hòu pò 厚朴 (Magnoliae Officinalis Cortex, officinal magnolia bark)
bàn xià 半夏 (Pinelliae Rhizoma, pinellia)
dàn zhú yè 淡竹叶 (Lophatheri Herba, lophatherum)
huá shí (滑石 (Talcum, talcum)
tōng cǎo 通草 (Tetrapanacis Medulla, rice-paper plant pith)
Plus:
zǐ wǎn 紫菀 (Asteris Radix, aster)
pí pá yè 枇杷叶 (Eriobotryae Folium, loquat leaf)

湿浊上泛

肺失宣降， 津液不行， 转化为湿， 停聚上焦， 常与热合， 形成上焦湿热证。可见恶寒发热， 咳嗽痰白， 身热不扬， 头身重痛， 胸闷脘痞， 舌苔淡黄厚腻等症。《温病纵横•湿热病》说: “上焦湿热证候， …是湿热邪气自口鼻而入， 侵袭于肺， 导致肺气宣发肃降失司， 卫外功能失常及水液代谢障碍的一类证候。” 治宜清热化湿， 宣肺除痰。方选《温病条辨》三仁汤（杏仁、白蔻仁、苡仁、厚朴、半夏、淡竹叶、滑石、通草）加紫菀、枇杷叶。

3.2.3 Phlegm-Rheum Collecting in the Lung

If the lung's diffusion and downbearing are impaired and the fluids do not move, they can transform into rheum and phlegm, which can create phlegm-rheum patterns. These manifest in panting and cough, copious clear thin phlegm that is white and foamy in appearance, fullness and oppression in the chest and diaphragm, dry mouth and thirst, a liking for hot drinks, a green-blue face, and cold limbs.

The chapter, "Various Symptoms of Phlegm-Rheum Disease" in the *Zhū Bìng Yuán Hòu Lùn* ("The Origin and Indicators of Disease") explains: "Phlegm-rheum is caused by qì block in the vessels and by stoppage of the fluids. Water-rheum and qì collect in the chest, bind together, and become phlegm." The "Section on Phlegm-Rheum" in the *Shèng Jì Zǒng Lù* ("Sages' Salvation Records") also explains:

> "Transformation of water is based on the diffusion and flow of qì in the vessels…When the flow of qì in the triple burner is rough and the vessel pathways are blocked, water-rheum collects and stagnates. Unable to diffuse and move, it gathers and forms phlegm-rheum. This causes a great variety of diseases." The reference in this source to water-rheum collecting and unable to diffuse clearly illumines the pathomechanism of impaired diffusion and downbearing of the lung with water collecting and transforming into rheum.

This condition is treated by warming the lung and transforming rheum, and by drying dampness and eliminating phlegm. The recommended formula is *líng gān wǔ wèi jiāng xīn bàn xià xìng rén tāng* (Poria, Licorice, Schisandra, Ginger, Asarum, Pinellia, Almond Seed Decoction) from the *Jīn Guì Yào Lüè* ("Essential Prescriptions of the Golden Coffer") with the addition of *guì zhī* (Cinnamomi Ramulus), *zǐ wǎn* (Asteris Radix), and *kuǎn dōng huā* (Farfarae Flos).

Líng Gān Wǔ Wèi Jiāng Xīn Bàn Xià Xìng Rén Tāng
苓甘五味姜辛半夏杏仁汤
(Poria, Licorice, Schisandra, Ginger, Asarum, Pinellia, and Almond Decoction)

fú líng 茯苓 (Poria, poria)
gān cǎo 甘草 (Glycyrrhizae Radix, licorice)
wǔ wèi zǐ 五味子 (Schisandrae Fructus, schisandra)
gān jiāng 干姜 (Zingiberis Rhizoma , dried ginger)
xì xīn 细辛 (Asari Radix, asarum)
bàn xià 半夏 (Pinelliae Rhizoma, pinellia)
xìng rén 杏仁 (Armeniacae Semen, almond)
Plus:
guì zhī 桂枝 (Cinnamomi Ramulus, cinnamon twig)
zǐ wǎn 紫菀 (Asteris Radix, aster)
kuǎn dōng huā 款冬花 (Farfarae Flos, coltsfoot)

痰饮停肺

若肺失宣降，津液不行，化饮成痰，可形成痰饮证，可见咳嗽气喘、痰多清稀、呈白色泡沫状、胸膈满闷、口干渴、喜热饮，面青肢冷等症状。《诸病源候论•痰饮病诸候》说："痰饮者，由气脉闭塞，津液不通，水饮气停在胸府，结而成痰。"《圣济总录•痰饮门》亦说："水之所化，凭气脉以宣流，…三焦气涩，脉道闭塞，则水饮停滞，不得宣行，聚成痰饮，为病多端。"文中"水饮停滞，不得宣行"即指肺失宣降，水停化饮的病机。治宜温肺化饮，燥湿除痰。方选《金匮要略》苓甘五味姜辛半夏杏仁汤（茯苓、五味、干姜、细辛、半夏、杏仁、甘草）加桂枝、紫菀、冬花。

3.2.4 Phlegm Turbidity Obstructing the Lung

When the lung's diffusion and downbearing are impaired, it is unable to regulate the waterways. The fluids are not distributed, but collect in the lung, where they transform into phlegm turbidity. Alternatively, this condition can be caused by the spleen's failure to move and transform, which disturbs the distribution of the fluids. As a result, they transform into dampness and form phlegm, which flows up into the lung and creates this condition. This is referred to by the expression, "the spleen is the source of phlegm formation; the lung is the receptacle that holds phlegm."

When phlegm turbidity arises, it forms pathological substances that collect and stagnate in the lung. These can in turn give rise to new pathological factors by further congesting lung qì and impairing the lung's diffusion and downbearing. This situation manifests in panting and cough, fullness and oppression in the chest and diaphragm, phlegm that is copious, white, and easy to expectorate, a thick slimy white tongue fur, and a slippery pulse.

The chapter, "Miscellaneous Pathoconditions; General Introduction and Combined Opinions on Major and Minor Issues in Phlegm-Rheum" in the *Píng Shì Jǐn Náng Mì Lù* ("Feng's Secret Record of the Brocade Pouch") explains:

> "The spleen is the source of phlegm formation...If the spleen is vacuous and unable to convey essence to the lung or move fluids down the waterways, the clear is difficult to upbear and the turbid is difficult to downbear. Both are retained in the middle, stagnate in the diaphragm, and form stasis and phlegm."

What is called "stagnating in the diaphragm" is a general reference to the chest and lung. Thus, when the spleen is unable to upbear the clear and downbear the turbid, the fluids do not move but collect in the center burner, flood up into the chest and lung, and impede the diffusion and downbearing of lung qì. Transforming into phlegm turbidity, this creates the pathomechanism of phlegm turbidity obstructing the lung.

The chapter, "Phlegm-Rheum" in the *Yī Zōng Bì Dú* ("Indispensable Medical Reading") further describes the clinical characteristics of damp phlegm:

> "When it is located in the spleen channel, it is called 'damp phlegm.' It manifests in a moderate pulse, yellow face, heaviness in the limbs, somnolence, abdominal distention and food stagnation, and slippery phlegm that is easy to expel."

This condition is treated by fortifying the spleen and drying dampness, and by downbearing qì and transforming phlegm. The recommended formula is *èr chén tāng* (Two Matured Ingredients Decoction) from the *Tài Píng Huì Mín Hé Jì Jú Fāng* (Tài-Píng Imperial Grace Pharmacy Formulas) with additions.

Èr Chén Tāng 二陈汤 (Two Matured Ingredients Decoction)
bàn xià 半夏 (Pinelliae Rhizoma, pinellia) *fú líng* 茯苓 (Poria, poria) *chén pí* 陈皮 (Citri Reticulatae Pericarpium, tangerine peel) *gān cǎo* 甘草 (Glycyrrhizae Radix, licorice) Plus: *xìng rén* 杏仁 (Armeniacae Semen, apricot kernel) *hòu pò* 厚朴 (Magnoliae Officinalis Cortex, officinal magnolia bark) *cāng zhú* 苍术 (Atractylodis Rhizoma, atractylodes) *yì yǐ rén* 薏苡仁 (Coicis Semen, coix) *zǐ sū zǐ* 紫苏子 (Perillae Fructus, perilla fruit)

痰浊阻肺

肺失宣降，不能通调水道，水津不布，停留于肺，可转化为痰浊。或由脾失健运，津液输布障碍，化湿生痰，上泛于肺而成，即所谓“脾为生痰之源，肺为贮痰之器。”痰浊生成，作为病理产物，停滞肺中，又可成为新的致病因素，进一步阻塞肺气，导致肺失宣降，引起咳嗽气喘、胸膈满闷、痰多色白易咯，苔白厚腻，脉滑等症。如《冯氏锦囊秘录•杂症•痰饮大小总论合参》说：“然脾为生痰之源，…惟脾虚不能致精于肺，下输水道，则清者难升，浊者难降，留中滞膈，瘀而成痰。”所谓“滞膈”是泛指胸肺，即脾不升清降浊，津液不行，停留于中焦，上泛于胸肺，阻碍肺气的宣降，转化为痰浊，形成痰浊阻肺的病机。《医宗必读•痰饮》云：“在脾经者，名曰湿痰，脉缓面黄肢体沉重，嗜卧不收，腹胀食滞，其痰滑而易出。”进一步阐述了湿痰的临床特征。治宜健脾燥湿，降气化痰。方选《和剂局方》二陈汤加杏仁、厚朴、苍术、苡仁、苏子。

3.2.5 Rheum Collecting in the Chest and Rib-Side

When the lung's diffusion and downbearing are impaired, it is unable to distribute and disperse the fluids. As a result, they gather and become rheum. When they collect in the region of the chest and rib-side, they become suspended rheum. The chapter, “Pulse Symptoms and Treatments of Phlegm-Rheum Cough” in the *Jīn Guì Yào Lüè* (“Essential Prescriptions of the Golden Coffer”) explains: “After drinking, water flows into the area below the rib-side and causes cough and spitting that induces pain. This is called suspended rheum.” The “Section on Cough,

Panting, and Phlegm-Rheum" in the *Yán Shì Jì Shēng Fāng* ("Yan's Remedies for Curing All People") states:

> "It is essential for the airways in the human body to be smooth. When they are smooth, the fluids flow freely and there will be absolutely no problem with phlegm-rheum. With improper regulation and containment however, the airways are blocked and water-rheum collects in the chest and diaphragm. There it binds and becomes phlegm, which causes disease."

This is a detailed analysis of the pathomechanism by which a deranged qì dynamic prevents qì from moving liquid. Instead, they collect in the chest and diaphragm and form phlegm-rheum. When rheum collects in the chest and rib-side, it obstructs the paths of the network vessels. Upbearing and downbearing by lung qì becomes abnormal and diffusion and downbearing are disturbed. This results in bulging in the chest and rib-side, distention, fullness, and pain, shortness of breath and hasty panting, cough possibly with pain when turning sides, a thin white tongue fur, and a stringlike pulse.

This condition is treated by attacking and expelling phlegm-rheum, and by rectifying qì and freeing the network vessels. The treatment method varies depending on the severity of water accumulation. For severe water accumulation, the recommended formula is *shí zǎo tāng* (Ten Jujubes Decoction) from the *Shāng Hán Lùn* ("On Cold Damage").

Shí Zǎo Tāng 十枣汤 (Ten Jujubes Decoction)
yuán huā 芫花 (Genkwa Flos, genkwa)
gān suì 甘遂 (Kansui Radix, kansui
dà zǎo 大枣 (Jujubae Fructus, jujube)

For relatively mild water accumulation, the recommended formula is *xiāng fù xuān fù huā tāng* (Cyperus and Inula Decoction) from the *Wēn Bìng Tiáo Bian* ("Systematized Identification of Warm Diseases") with additions.

Xiāng Fù Xuān Fù Huā Tāng 香附旋覆花汤 (Cyperus and Inula Decoction)
xiāng fù 香附 (Cyperi Rhizoma, cyperus)
xuán fù huā 旋覆花 (Inulae Flos, inula flower)
zǐ sū zǐ 紫苏子 (Perillae Fructus, perilla fruit)
bàn xià 半夏 (Pinelliae Rhizoma, pinellia)
fú líng 茯苓 (Poria, poria)
chén pí 陈皮 (Citri Reticulatae Pericarpium, tangerine peel)
yì yǐ rén 薏苡仁 (Coicis Semen, coix)
Plus:

yù jīn 郁金 (Curcumae Radix, curcuma)
chái hú 柴胡 (Bupleuri Radix, bupleurum)
chì sháo 芍药 (Paeoniae Radix Rubra, red peony)
tíng lì zǐ 葶苈子 (Lepidii/Descurainiae Semen, lepidium/descurainiae)

饮停胸胁

肺失宣降，不能布散津液，聚而为饮，停留于胸胁之间，成为悬饮.《金匮要略•痰饮咳嗽病脉证并治》说："饮后水流在胁下．咳唾引痛，谓之悬饮．"《重订严氏济生方•咳喘痰饮门》云："人之气道贵乎顺，顺则津液流通，决无痰饮之患．调摄失宜，气道闭塞，水饮停于胸膈，结而成痰，其为病也．" 详细分析了气机失调，气不行津，停留胸膈，引起痰饮的病机．饮停胸胁，络道被阻，肺气升降失常，宣降失司，则胸胁彭隆，胀满疼痛，呼吸气短喘促，咳嗽或转侧牵引作痛，苔薄白，脉弦．治宜攻逐水饮，理气通络．治疗根据积水轻重，方法不同．积水重者，选《伤寒论》十枣汤（芫花、甘遂、大枣）.

积水较少， 选《温病条辨》香附旋覆花汤（香附、旋覆花、苏子、半夏、茯苓、陈皮， 苡仁）加郁金、柴胡、赤芍、葶苈子。

Literature Review of Non-Distribution of Fluids

📖 *Jīn Guì Yào Lüè* ("Essential Prescriptions of the Golden Coffer"), "Pulse Symptoms and Treatments of Water Qì Disease"

> "In wind water, the pulse is naturally floating, and the external signs are joint pain and aversion to wind. When the inch opening pulse is sunken and slippery, and there is water qì in the center, the head and face are swollen and enlarged, and there is heat, this is called 'wind water.' One sees slight swelling of the eye nest, as [in one] newly arisen from sleep; the neck pulse stirs, and there is frequent coughing. When you press the hands or feet, they pit but do not spring back. [All this constitutes] wind water."

This quotation describes how external evil assailing the lung impairs the lung's diffusion and downbearing and the distribution of fluids, which leads to wind water. In addition, it emphasizes prior swelling of the head and face as the most important characteristic among the pulses and signs.

📖 *Wài Tái Mì Yào* ("Essential Secrets from Outside the Metropolis"), "Xǔ Rén-zé's Formulas for Treating Cough"

> "Cough due to rheum qì occurs when ingested fluids collect in the chest, and water qì surges upward into the lung. When the lung receives this qì, it causes cough. If it is not eliminated for a long time, it gradually becomes water qì."

This quotation describes how cough is formed by water-rheum invading the upper body and collecting in the lung, which impairs the lung's diffusion and downbearing and causes counterflow qì ascent. As water rheum is unable to diffuse, it creates water swelling.

📖 *Lín Zhèng Zhǐ Nán Yī Àn* ("A Clinical Guide with Case Histories"), "Dampness" A case history

> "Damp-warmth obstructing lung defense manifested in a sore pharynx and impediment in the instep. When I cleared the upper burner, dampness left and qì was naturally harmonized. I used *huá shí* (Talcum), tender lophatherum leaf *zhú yè xīn* (Lophatheri Folium Immaturum), *lián qiào* (Forsythiae Fructus), *jié gěng* (Platycodonis Radix), *shè gān* (Belamcandae Rhizoma), and *lú gēn* (Phragmitis Rhizoma)."

This quotation discusses a case where an external contraction of warm-heat disease evil prevented lung-defense from diffusing, inhibited lung qì, and impaired the distribution of fluids, with the result that damp warmth evil collected in the upper burner. Dr. Yè effectively treated this condition by clearing and diffusing damp heat in the upper burner.

📖 *Wēn Bìng Tiáo Bian* ("Systematized Identification of Warm Diseases"), "Chapter on the Lower Burner"

> "Latent summerheat or damp warmth can accumulate as propping rheum and become suspended under the rib-side. This creates a great amount of rib-side pain, which is precisely the sign of water in the lung that the *Jīn Guì Yào Lüe* ("Essential Prescriptions of the Golden Coffer") treats with *shí zǎo tāng* (Ten Jujubes Decoction). The reason for that approach is that an enduring accumulation of internal water cannot be dealt with in any other way than by stern attack. My own reason [for a different approach] is that seasonal evil, when it just begins to contend with internal water, is not yet rooted securely. You therefore do not need to employ the drastic nature of *shí zǎo tāng* (Ten Jujubes Decoction), but can use only *xiāng fù* (Cyperi Rhizoma) and *xuán fù huā* (Inulae Flos) to free the lung network vessels and expel the rheum under the rib-side."

This quotation describes the pathomechanism and treatment method for an external invasion of seasonal evil that impairs the lung's diffusion and downbearing and causes water-rheum to collect in the chest and rib-side.

文献评述

《金匮要略•水气病脉证并治曰: : “风水， 其脉自浮， 外证骨节疼痛， 恶风。…寸口脉沉滑者， 中有水气， 面目肿大， 有热， 名曰风水。视人之目窠上微肿， 如蚕新卧起状， 其颈脉动， 时时咳， 按其手足上， 陷而不起者， 风水。” 论述外邪袭肺， 肺失宣降， 水津失布， 引起风水， 及以头面先肿为主要特征的脉证。

《外台秘要•许仁则疗咳嗽方》曰: “饮气嗽者， 由所饮之物， 停滞在胸， 水气上冲， 冲入于肺， 肺得此气便成嗽， 久而不除， 渐成水气。” 论述水饮上犯， 停聚于肺， 肺失宣降， 气上逆而成咳嗽; 水饮不得宣散， 而成水肿。

《临证指南医案•湿》某案曰: “湿温阻于肺卫， 咽痛， 足跗痹痛， 当清上焦， 湿走气自和。飞滑石、竹叶心、连翘、桔梗、射干、芦根。” 此为外感温热病邪， 肺卫失宣， 肺气不利， 水津失布， 湿温之邪停留上焦所致病案， 叶氏用清宣上焦湿热而获效。

《温病条辨•下焦篇》曰: “伏暑湿温， 积留支饮， 悬于胁下， 而成胁痛之证甚多， 即金匮水在肝而用十枣汤之证。彼因里水久积， 非峻攻不可。此因时令之邪， 与里水新搏, 其根不固，不必用十枣之太峻，只以香附、旋覆花善通肝络而逐胁下之饮。” 阐述时令之邪外侵，肺失宣降，水饮停于胸胁的病机和治法。

Summary of Non-Distribution of the Fluids

1. Internal Collection of Water Qì

   Rapid disease onset; severe swelling that is most pronounced in the head and face and upper half of the body; short voidings of scant urine.

2. Damp Turbidity Flooding Upward

   Aversion to cold and heat effusion, cough with white phlegm, unsurfaced generalized heat, heavy and aching head and body, oppression in the chest and glomus in the stomach duct, thick and slimy pale yellow tongue fur.

3. Phlegm-Rheum Collecting in the Lung

   Panting and cough, copious clear thin phlegm that is white and foamy in appearance, fullness and oppression in the chest and diaphragm, dry mouth and thirst, liking for hot drinks, green-blue face and cold limbs.

4. Phlegm Turbidity Obstructing the Lung
   Panting and cough, fullness and oppression in the chest and diaphragm, copious white phlegm that is easy to expectorate, thick slimy white tongue fur, slippery pulse.
5. Rheum Collecting in the Chest and Rib-Side
   Bulging in the chest and rib-side; distention, fullness, and pain; shortness of breath and hasty panting; cough possibly with pain from turning sides, thin white tongue fur, stringlike pulse.

津液不布

水气内停
   发病急，多见头面、上半身肿甚，小便短少。
湿浊上泛
   恶寒发热，咳嗽痰白，身热不扬，头身重痛，胸闷脘痞，舌苔淡黄厚腻。
痰饮停肺
   咳嗽气喘、痰多清稀、呈白色泡沫状、胸膈满闷、口干渴、喜热饮，面青肢冷。
痰浊阻肺
   咳嗽气喘、胸膈满闷、痰多色白易咯，苔白厚腻，脉滑。
饮停胸胁
   胸胁彭隆，胀满疼痛，呼吸气短喘促，咳嗽或转侧牵引作痛，苔薄白，脉弦。

3.3 Qì and Blood Depression

The lung is located above the diaphragm and in close proximity to the heart. The heart governs the blood and vessels; the lung governs the qì of the entire body. All qì in the viscera and bowels, channels and network vessels is perfused by lung qì. The lung assembles the hundred vessels, and the blood vessels of the whole body all meet in the lung. Lung qì is also closely involved in the movement of blood and assists the heart in moving blood. Once lung qì is obstructed and diffusion and depurative downbearing break down, this can lead to the pathomechanism of lung qì depression and obstruction with inhibited blood flow.

The chapter, "Needling Divisions, True [Qì] and Evil [Qì]" in the *Líng Shū* ("The Magic Pivot") explains: "When ancestral qì fails to descend, the blood inside the vessels leaves, congeals, and stops." Ancestral qì means precisely the great qì inside the lung. Qì is the commander of blood and makes blood move. "If qì does not move in one breath, neither does blood."

The section on blood in the "Chapter on the Internal Landscape" in the *Dōng Yī Bǎo Jiàn* ("Precious Mirror of Eastern Medicine") explains that a derangement of lung qì can lead to inhibition in the blood vessels. If lung qì fails to move, blood collects inside the lung, and the blood vessels suffer from stasis obstruction. This can manifest in such symptoms as panting, cough, and shortness of breath, and in welling-abscess or distention of the lung.

It is treated by supplementing qì and quickening blood, and by downbearing qì and calming panting. The recommended formula is *bǔ fèi tāng* (Lung-Supplementing Decoction) from the *Yǒng Lèi Líng Fāng* ("Previously Published Formulas for the Benefit of All Posterity") with additions.

Bǔ Fèi Tāng 补肺汤 (Lung-Supplementing Decoction)
rén shēn 人参 (Ginseng Radix, ginseng)
huáng qí 黄芪 (Astragali Radix, astragalus)
shú dì huáng 熟地黄 (Rehmanniae Radix Praeparata, cooked rehmannia)
wǔ wèi zǐ 五味子 (Schisandrae Fructus, schisandra)
zǐ wǎn 紫菀 (Asteris Radix, aster)
sāng bái pí 桑白皮 (Mori Cortex, mulberry root bark)
Plus:
dāng guī 当归 (Angelicae Sinensis Radix, Chinese angelica)
táo rén 桃仁 (Persicae Semen, peach kernel)
xìng rén 杏仁 (Armeniacae Semen, apricot kernel)
hòu pò 厚朴 (Magnoliae Officinalis Cortex, officinal magnolia bark)
zǐ sū zǐ 紫苏子 (Perillae Fructus, perilla fruit)

If blood stagnates in the network vessels of the heart as a result of lung qì failing to move, you will see symptoms of heart vessel obstruction, such as oppression and stifling pain in the chest, heart palpitations, and fearful throbbing. This condition is treated by supplementing the center and boosting qì, and by quickening blood and freeing impediment. The recommended formula is *rén shēn tāng* (Ginseng Decoction) from the *Jīn Guì Yào Lüè* ("Essential Prescriptions of the Golden Coffer") with additions.

Rén Shēn Tāng 人参汤 (Ginseng Decoction)
rén shēn 人参 (Ginseng Radix, ginseng)
bái zhú 白术 (Atractylodis Macrocephalae Rhizoma, white atractylodes)
gān jiāng 干姜 (Zingiberis Rhizoma, dried ginger)
gān cǎo 甘草 (Glycyrrhizae Radix, licorice)

Plus:
chuān xiōng 川芎 (Chuanxiong Rhizoma, chuanxiong)
dāng guī 当归 (Angelicae Sinensis Radix, Chinese angelica)
sān qī 三七 (Notoginseng Radix, notoginseng)
yù jīn 郁金 (Curcumae Radix, curcuma)

When evil qì lies depressed in the lung and blocks its action and when phlegm turbidity congests the lung, this impairs diffusion and downbearing. This can affect the heart and by inhibiting heart blood, cause dual disease of the heart and lung. The result is hasty panting and oppression in the chest, cough and ejection of phlegm-drool, heart palpitation and shortness of breath, and dark purple lips and face. This condition is treated by supplementing and boosting the heart and lung, and by quickening blood and transforming phlegm. The recommended formula is *bǎo yuán tāng* (Origin-Preserving Decoction) from the *Jǐng Yuè Quán Shū* ("Jǐng-Yuè's Complete Compendium") in combination with *guā lóu xiè bái bàn xià tāng* (Trichosanthes, Chinese Chive, and Pinellia Decoction) from the *Jīn Guì Yào Lüe* ("Essential Prescriptions of the Golden Coffer") with additions.

Bǎo Yuán Tāng 保元汤 (Origin-Preserving Decoction)
rén shēn 人参 (Ginseng Radix, ginseng) *huáng qí* 黄耆 (Astragali Radix, astragalus) *guì zhī* 桂枝 (Cinnamomi Ramulus, cinnamon twig) *gān cǎo* 甘草 (Glycyrrhizae Radix, licorice)

Guā Lóu Xiè Bái Bàn Xià Tāng 栝楼薤白半夏汤 (Trichosanthes, Chinese Chive, and Pinellia Decoction)
guā lóu 栝楼 (Trichosanthis Fructus, trichosanthes) *xiè bái* 薤白 (Allii Macrostemonis Bulbus, Chinese chive) *bàn xià* 半夏 (Pinelliae Rhizoma, pinellia) *báijiǔ* 白酒 (Granorum Spiritus Incolor, white liquor) Plus: *xìng rén* 杏仁 (Armeniacae Semen, apricot kernel) *hòu pò* 厚朴 (Magnoliae Officinalis Cortex, officinal magnolia bark) *táo rén* 桃仁 (Persicae Semen, peach kernel) *dāng guī* 当归 (Angelicae Sinensis Radix, Chinese angelica)

In externally contracted warm-heat disease in which warm evil invades the lung and impairs diffusion and downbearing, if the disease of the qì affects the blood, it can easily cause pathologies in the heart and pericardium. "Yè Xiāng-Yán's Chapter on Externally Contracted Damp-Heat Disease" in the *Wēn Rè Jīng Wěi* ("Warp and Weft of Warm Heat") explains: "Because of the close relationship between lung and heart, lung heat is most likely to pass to the heart." This quotation shows why the pathomechanism of "warm evil contraction in the upper body, initial invasion of the lung, then abnormal passage to the pericardium" is a common pathology in warm disease. It is treated by clearing the heart and opening the orifices. Taking the circumstances into account, such formulas as *niú huáng qīng xīn wán* (Bovine Bezoar Heart-Clearing Pill), *ān gōng niú huáng wán* (Peaceful Palace Bovine Bezoar Pill), *zhì bǎo dān* (Supreme Jewel Elixir), or *zǐ xuě dān* (Purple Snow Elixir) are used.

Niú Huáng Qīng Xīn Wán 牛黄清心丸 (Bovine Bezoar Heart-Clearing Pill)
niú huáng 牛黄 (Bovis Calculus, bovine bezoar)
zhū shā 朱砂 (Cinnabaris, cinnabar)
huáng lián 黄连 (Coptidis Rhizoma, coptis)
huáng qín 黄芩 (Scutellariae Radix, scutellaria)
zhī zǐ 栀子 (Gardeniae Fructus, gardenia)
yù jīn 郁金 (Curcumae Radix, curcuma)

Ān Gōng Niú HuángWán 安宫牛黄丸 (Peaceful Palace Bovine Bezoar Pill)
niú huáng 牛黄 (Bovis Calculus, bovine bezoar)
xī jiǎo 犀角 (Cornu Rhinoceri, rhinoceros horn)
yù jīn 郁金 (Tuber Curcumae, curcuma)
huáng qín 黄芩 (Scutellariae Radix, scutellaria)
huáng lián 黄连 (Rhizoma Coptidis, coptis)
zhī zǐ 栀子 (Gardeniae Fructus, gardenia)
zhū shā 朱砂 (Cinnabaris, cinnabar)
xióng huáng 雄黄 (Realgar, realgar)
zhēn zhū 珍珠(Margarita, pearl)
shè xiāng 麝香 (Moschus, musk)
bīng piàn 冰片(Borneolum, borneol)

Zhì Bǎo Dān 至宝丹 (Supreme Jewel Elixir)
xī jiǎo 犀角(Cornu Rhinoceri, rhinoceros horn)
niú huáng 牛黄 (Bovis Calculus, bovine bezoar)
dài mào 玳瑁 (Eretmochelydis Carapax, hawksbill shell)
bīng piàn 冰片 (Borneolum, borneol)
shè xiāng 麝香 (Moschus, musk)
ān xī xiāng 安息香 (Benzoinum, benzoin)
zhū shā 朱砂 (Cinnabaris, cinnabar)
hǔ pò 琥珀 (Succinum, amber)
xióng huáng 雄黄 (Realgar, realgar)

Zǐ Xuě Dān 紫雪丹 (Purple Snow Elixir)
shí gāo 石膏 (Gypsum Fibrosum, gypsum)
hán shuǐ shí 寒水石 (Gypsum seu Calcitum, glauberite)
huá shí 滑石 (Talcum, talcum)
xī jiǎo 犀角 (Cornu Rhinoceri, rhinoceros horn)
líng yáng jiǎo 羚羊角 (Saigae Tataricae Cornu, antelope horn)
shè xiāng 麝香 (Moschus, musk)
xuán shēn 玄参 (Scrophulariae Radix, scrophularia)
cí shí 磁石 (Magnetitum, loadstone)
shēng má 升麻 (Cimicifugae Rhizoma, cimicifuga)
zhì gān cǎo 炙甘草 (Glycyrrhizae Radix Praeparata, mix-fried licorice)
qīng mù xiāng 青木香 (Aristolochiae Radix, aristolochia root [vladimiria])
dīng xiāng 丁香 (Caryophylli Flos, clove)
zhū shā 朱砂 (Cinnabaris, cinnabar)
máng xiāo 芒硝 (Natrii Sulfas, mirabilite)
xiāo shí 硝石 (Nitrum, niter)
huáng jīn 黄金 (Aurum, gold)

气血郁滞

肺居膈上, 与心脏相近, 心主血脉, 肺主一身之气, 凡脏腑经络之气, 皆由肺气所宣. 肺朝百脉, 全身血脉皆会聚于肺, 肺气与血液运行密切相关, 有助心行血的作用. 肺气一旦阻滞, 宣发肃降失职, 则可导致肺气郁阻, 血流不畅的病机. 如《灵枢•刺节真邪篇》说: "宗气不下, 脉中之血, 离凝而留止." 宗气即肺中的大气, 气为血帅, 气令血行, "气有一息不运, 则血有一息不行." (《东医宝鉴•内景篇•血》) 说明肺气逆乱, 可致血脉不利. 若肺气不行, 血停肺中, 血脉瘀阻, 可见咳喘气短、肺痈肺胀等症. 治宜补气活血, 降气平喘. 方选《永类钤方》补肺汤（人参、黄芪、熟地、五味、紫菀、桑白皮）加当归、桃仁、杏仁、厚朴、苏子;

若肺气不行，血滞心脏络脉，可见胸闷憋痛，心悸怔忡等心脉痹阻等症。治宜补中益气，活血通痹，方选《金匮要略》人参汤（人参、白术、干姜、甘草）加川芎、当归、三七、郁金;

若邪气闭郁，痰浊壅遏，肺失宣降，影响及心，心血不畅，可致心肺同病，则为喘促胸闷，咳吐痰涎，心悸气短，面唇紫暗等症。治宜补益心肺，活血化痰。方选《景岳全书》保元汤（人参、黄芪、桂枝、甘草）合《金匮要略》栝蒌薤白半夏汤（栝蒌实、薤白、半夏、白酒）加杏仁、厚朴、桃仁、当归。

在外感温热病中，温邪犯肺，宣降失职，由气及血，易引起心及心包的病变。如《温热经纬•叶香岩外感温热病篇》说："肺与心相通，故肺热最易传心。"表现为温病的传变中常见"温邪上受，首先犯肺，逆传心包"的病机。治宜清心开窍。可酌情选用牛黄清心丸、安宫牛黄丸、至宝丹、紫雪丹等方药。

Literature Review of Qì and Blood Depression

📖 *Jīn Guì Yào Lüè* ("Essential Prescriptions of the Golden Coffer"), "Pulse Symptoms and Treatments of Lung Wilting, Lung Welling-Abscess, Cough, and Qì Ascent"

"Wind damages the skin and body hair; heat damages the blood and vessels. Wind abides in the lung. A person affected by wind presents with cough, dry mouth, panting and fullness, dry pharynx without thirst, copious turbid and foamy spittle, and frequent quivering with cold. Because of excess heat, blood congeals and stagnates, amasses and binds, and forms welling-abscesses with pus and gruel-like vomit. In the initial budding stage, this can be stemmed, but when pus forms, the result is death."

This quotation describes the disease cause and pathology of lung welling-abscess, caused by static blood binding with evil heat and congesting the lung.

📖 *Xuè Zhèng Lùn* ("On Blood Patterns"), "Cough"

"The pathways of qì in the human body must not become congested! If there is static blood in them, it impedes them and impairs upbearing and downbearing. For this reason, congestion causes cough. Qì congestion means water congestion, because qì means water. When water is congested, it causes phlegm-rheum. When phlegm-rheum is obstructed by static blood, it surges even further into the lung channel. When sitting or standing, the lung functions as a cover and the static blood drops into the lower body. In that case, the pathways of qì are not yet hampered too severely and the cough is therefore also not severe. When lying down, the static blood reverses course and adds to the congestion. The lobes of the lung are stretched even further which makes them yet more difficult to constrain. This is the reason for propped breathing with inability to lie down.

If you treat water-rheum surging into the lung with *tíng lì dà zào tāng* (Descurainia and Jujube Decoction), you are employing the method of treating phlegm, but not the method of treating stasis. You must beware that the phlegm-water congestion is caused by static blood. When you simply dispel static blood, phlegm and water will disperse on their own. Thus, *dài dǐ dàng wán* (Substitute Dead-On Pill) is suitable, with the addition of *fú líng* (Poria) and *bàn xià* (Pinelliae Rhizoma). In mild cases, use *xuè fǔ zhú yū tāng* (House of Blood Stasis-Expelling Decoction), with the addition of lepidium/descurainiae *tíng lì zǐ* (Lepidii/Descurainiae Semen)."

This quotation describes the special features of the pathomechanism by which static blood collecting in the lung impedes the qì dynamic, forms phlegm-rheum, and leads to cough and counterflow with propped breathing and inability to lie down.

文献评述

《金匮要略•肺痿肺痈咳嗽上气病脉证治》曰: : "风伤皮毛，热伤血脉。风舍于肺，其人则咳，口干喘满，咽燥不渴，多唾浊沫，时时振寒。热之所过，血为之凝滞，蓄结痈脓，吐如米粥。始萌可救，脓成则死。"论述了瘀血与邪热相互结合，壅塞于肺，形成肺痈的病因及病理变化。

《血证论•咳嗽》曰: : "盖人身气道不可有塞滞，内有瘀血则阻碍气道不得升降，是以壅而为咳。气壅即水壅，气即水故也。水壅即为痰饮。痰饮为瘀血所阻，则益冲犯肺经，坐立则肺覆，瘀血亦下坠，其气道尚无大碍，故咳亦不甚。卧则瘀血翻转，更为阻塞，肺叶又张，愈难敛戢，是以倚息不得卧也。若照水饮冲肺，用葶苈大枣汤，是得其治饮之法，而未得治瘀之法矣。须知痰水之壅，由瘀血使然，但祛瘀血，则痰水自消，宜代抵当丸，加云茯苓法半夏。轻则用血府逐瘀汤，加葶苈苏子。"论述瘀血停肺，阻碍气机，化生痰饮，引起咳逆倚息不得卧的病机特点。

Summary of Qì and Blood Depression

1. Blood Collecting in the Lung

   Panting, cough, and shortness of breath; welling-abscess and distention of the lung.

2. Stasis Obstruction of the Heart Vessels

   Oppression and stifling pain in the chest; heart palpitations and fearful throbbing.

3. Heart and Lung Sharing a Disease

   Hasty panting and oppression in the chest; cough and ejection of phlegm-drool; heart palpitation and shortness of breath; dark purple face and lips.

4. Warmth Evil Invading the Lung

   Abnormal passage to the pericardium: Clouded spirit and delirious speech.

气血郁滞
血停肺中——咳喘气短，肺痈肺胀。
心脉瘀阻——胸闷憋痛，心悸怔忡。
心肺同病——喘促胸闷，咳吐痰涎，心悸气短，面唇紫暗。
温邪犯肺——逆传心包——神昏谵语。

Repeated impairment of lung diffusion and depurative downbearing can influence the lung's function of governing qì; wearing it down over a long period of time, it can lead to consumption of lung qì. Alternatively, it can influence the lung's function of engendering qì. When the formation of ancestral qì is reduced, it can also induce the pathomechanism of lung qì vacuity, leading in severe cases to vacuity of qì in the whole body. If the yáng evils of wind, dryness, summerheat, and heat assail it, or if the evils of cold or dampness or pathological substances collect in the lung, become depressed, and transform into fire, this can impair the lung's diffusion and downbearing and cause internal blazing of fire heat. This is likely to damage yīn humor and can also induce the pathomechanism of lung yīn vacuity.

肺的宣发肃降反复失常，影响肺的主气功能，日久消磨，可致肺气耗损；或影响肺的生气功能，宗气生成减少，均可引起肺气虚的病机发生，甚至引起全身之气虚弱。若受风、燥、暑、热等阳邪侵犯，或寒湿之邪及病理产物停肺，郁而化火，导致肺失宣降，火热内炽，易伤阴液，又可引起肺阴虚的病机.

PART TWO

Pathomechanisms of Lung Vacuity

Lung Vacuity

While the majority of lung pathomechanisms are marked by repletion, quite a few are associated with vacuity. Lung vacuity refers to the pathological changes that manifest when the lung's functions are weakened. This happens when the lung suffers the effect of a variety of pathogenic factors, such as the passage and transmutation of diseases from other bowels and viscera, excessive strength of pathogenic factors, or a reduction of right qì from a prolonged disease process. Any of these can harm the physiological functions of the lung and induce the pathomechanism of lung vacuity.

The earliest description of lung vacuity is found in the *Huáng Dì Nèi Jīng* ("The Yellow Emperor's Inner Canon"). "The Jade Swivel Treatise on True Visceral Pulses" in the *Sù Wèn* ("Plain Questions") explains: "[Lung] deficiency causes panting, breathing with shortage of qì and coughing, in the case of qì ascent with [coughing of] blood, and pathologic sounds in the lower body." In this source, deficiency refers to lung qì vacuity.

The *Zhōng Zàng Jīng* ("Central Treasury Canon") discusses the pathomechanisms of lung disease by dividing them into vacuity and repletion and directly mentions the pathomechanism of lung vacuity. The chapter, "Discussing the Pulses and Patterns of Vacuity and Repletion, Cold and Heat, Life and Death, and Favorable and Unfavorable Shifts in Lung Disease" in this text explains:

> "[Lung] vacuity results in engenderment of cold, breathing with coughing, and disinhibition in the lower body, in shortage of qì and of bodily strength, and in increased sensation of sorrow."
>
> "Vacuity results in inability to breathe, decreased hearing and dry throat, panting and cough with qì ascent, and shoulder and back pain."

The *Zhū Bìng Yuán Hòu Lùn* ("The Origin and Indicators of Disease"), *Qiān Jīn Yào Fāng* ("A Thousand Gold Pieces Prescriptions"), *Shèng Jì Zǒng Lù* ("Sages' Salvation Records"), and *Yán Shì Jì Shēng Fāng* ("Yan's Remedies for Curing All People") also contain descriptions of the pathomechanism of lung vacuity. During the Jīn-Yuán period, Zhū Dān-Xī explained in the chapter, "Panting" in the *Mài Yīn Zhèng Zhì* ("Pulses, Causes, Patterns and Treatment"): "Lung vacuity invariably manifests in dry throat with no liquid and in shortage of qì and insufficiency in breathing." All the above texts laid a solid foundation for the pathomechanism of lung vacuity.

When scanning the historical records, most sources emphasize lung qì vacuity and lung yīn vacuity in their discussions and mention yáng vacuity less frequently. More recently, the objective existence of the pathomechanism of lung yáng vacuity has been discussed repeatedly and has gradually become widely accepted. For a long time the belief has been that lung blood vacuity is extremely rare, since the blood vessels of the whole body all meet in the lung and the lung is therefore full of blood. However, some publications have recently touched upon the fact that when lung blood is vacuous and fails to moisten, the lung's functions are reduced, which can result in the symptoms of panting and cough. Thereby they have illustrated the putative existence of the pathomechanism of lung blood vacuity. However, since these discussions do not go into great depth, they have not yet succeeded in gaining wide-spread acceptance.

肺虚的病机

肺病的病机除大量属实外， 还存在不少属虚的病机。肺虚是指肺的功能虚衰所表现的病机变化。当肺受到各种致病因素的作用， 或由于其它脏腑疾病的传变， 或致病因素过强， 或病程日久正气受损， 都会导致肺的生理功能受到损害， 引起肺虚的病机变化。早在《黄帝内经》中已有关于肺虚病机的论述。如《素问•玉机真藏论》说: "其不及则令人喘， 呼吸少气而咳， 上气见咳血， 下闻病声。" 其不及， 即指肺气虚。《中藏经》把肺病病机按虚实分论， 直接提出肺虚的病机 。该书《论肺脏虚实寒热生死逆顺脉证》说: 肺 "虚则寒生咳息利下， 少气力， 多悲感。" "虚则不能息， 耳重嗌干， 喘咳上气， 肩背痛。" 其后《诸病源候论》，《千金要方》，《圣济总录》《济生方》等都有关于肺虚病机的阐述， 金元时代朱丹溪《脉因证治•喘》也说: "肺虚者， 必咽干无津， 少气不足以息也。" 以上均为肺虚的病机奠定了坚实的基础。纵观历代文献， 侧重讨论肺的气虚， 阴虚者多， 较少提及肺的阳虚。经过近年来反复讨论， 肺阳虚的病机客观存在， 逐渐已被公认。关于肺的血虚， 长期以来， 认为周身血脉均会聚于肺， 肺中血液充足， 故肺的血虚， 极为罕见。不过， 近来亦有人论及肺血虚亏， 失于滋润， 肺的功能减弱， 可引起咳嗽气喘之症， 说明肺血虚的病机理当存在。只是由于讨论不太深入， 还未得到大家普遍的公认。

Chapter Four

Lung Qì Vacuity

The earliest reference to the pathomechanism of lung qì vacuity is found in the *Huáng Dì Nèi Jīng* ("The Yellow Emperor's Inner Canon"). The "Treatise on Comparative Exuberance and Debilitation" in the *Sù Wèn* ("Plain Questions"), for example, mentions the pathomechanism by which lung qì vacuity prevents storage of the corporeal soul, which results in spirit-mind disquietude. "Lung qì vacuity gives people visions in their dreams of white things, of beheaded corpses and blood flowing chaotically, and of soldiers and warfare." The chapter, "Methods of Treating Visceral Qì in Accordance with the Seasons" in the *Sù Wèn* ("Plain Questions") describes the pathomechanism of lung qì vacuity causing cough and panting: "Lung disease manifests in qì counterflow panting and cough and in shoulder and back pain …Vacuity results in shortage of qì with inability to catch one's breath, deafness, and dry throat." The *Líng Shū* ("The Magic Pivot") also describes in detail how lung qì vacuity leads to irregularities in the respiratory functions. The chapter, "The Spirit" in the *Líng Shū* ("The Magic Pivot") explains: "Lung qì vacuity results in nasal congestion and inhibition, and in shortage of qì." The chapter, "The Channel Vessels" also explains: "Qì vacuity results in cold shoulders and back, shortage of qì preventing normal breathing, and changes in the color of urine."

In subsequent generations, many texts elaborated on the pathomechanism of lung qì vacuity. For example, the *Zhū Bìng Yuán Hòu Lùn* ("The Origin and Indicators of Disease"), the *Yī Xué Rù Mén* ("The Gateway to Medicine"), the *Míng Yī Zhǐ Zhǎng* ("Illuminating Medicine in the Palm of Your Hand"), and the *Jǐng Yuè Quán Shū* ("Jǐng-Yuè's Complete Compendium") comprehensively explored how lung qì vacuity leads to disorders of external defense, disturbances in the fluid metabolism, and impaired nourishment to the viscera and bowels. The contributions of their work have increased and perfected our understanding of the pathomechanism of lung qì vacuity.

In sum, lung qì vacuity can be caused by enduring cough and panting, excessive taxation fatigue, insufficient formation or constitutional endowment, debility in old age, and lack of or inappropriate treatment. The pathomechanism of lung qì vacuity can be differentiated into such aspects as forceless breathing, insecurity of external defense, stoppage of the fluids, failure of the upper body to control the lower body, debilitation of ancestral qì, and lung qì verging on desertion.

肺气虚

最早提出肺气虚病机的是《黄帝内经》。如《素问•方盛衰论》提到肺气虚不能藏魄而致神志不安的病机:“肺气虚则使人梦白物, 见人斩血藉藉, 得其时, 则梦见兵战。”《素问•藏气法时论》阐述了肺气虚引起咳喘的病机:“肺病者, 喘咳气逆, 肩背痛, …虚则气少不能报息, 耳聋嗌干。”《灵枢》对肺气虚引起呼吸功能失调的病机作了深入论述。《灵枢•本神篇》说:“肺气虚, 则鼻塞不利, 少气。”《灵枢•经脉篇》又说:“气虚, 则肩背寒, 少气不足以息, 尿色变。”后世对肺气虚的病机代有发挥。如《诸病源候论》、《医学入门》、《明医指掌》、《景岳全书》等对肺气虚引起卫外功能失调、水液代谢障碍、脏腑失养等病机作了全面探讨,使对肺气虚病机的认识日臻完善。概括起来, 久病咳喘, 劳倦过度, 生化、禀赋不足, 年老体衰, 失治误治, 为引起肺气虚的病因。肺气虚的病机可分为呼吸无力, 卫外不固, 津液不行, 上不制下, 宗气衰少, 肺气欲脱等几个方面。

4.1 Forceless Breathing

The lung governs qì. It is in charge of breathing, exhales the old and inhales the new, and carries out the exchange of gas. If lung qì is damaged by a variety of causes, it debilitates organ functions and weakens respiratory strength. This can cause a series of manifestations of lung qì vacuity and weakness.

When lung qì is vacuous, it lacks strength to free the nasal orifices. This causes nasal congestion and poor sense of smell, because lung qì flowing to the nose causes the lung to be harmonized and able to discern good and bad smells. “Lung qì vacuity results in nasal congestion and inhibition” (*Líng Shū* (“The Magic Pivot”), “The Spirit”). When lung qì is vacuous, it is unable to promote the contraction and expansion of the lung’s lobes and to carry out diffusion and depurative downbearing. Instead, it moves upward in counterflow. This manifests in symptoms like cough with counterflow and snivel or with panting and lack of strength, low voice and qì timidity, and loss of voice, which are aggravated by movement.

The chapter "On the Pulses and Patterns of Vacuity and Repletion, Cold and Heat, Life and Death, and Favorable and Unfavorable Shifts in the Lung" in the *Zhōng Zàng Jīng* ("Central Treasury Canon") explains: "Vacuity results in lack of strength and hasty panting, distention in the left rib-side, and shortness of breath when speaking." When lung qì is vacuous and breathing is forceless, the exhaled and inhaled qì is reduced in every breath. To satisfy the demand for qì in the whole body, the lung is forced to accelerate the frequency of breathing, and the patient feels unable to catch their breath. This manifests in dyspnea and is called shortness of breath.

The chapter, "Panting Patterns" in the *Míng Yī Zhǐ Zhǎng* ("Illuminating Medicine in the Palm of Your Hand") states this precisely: "When lung qì is too vacuous, qì is unable to distribute breath, respiration is not continuous, and exhalation is greater than inhalation. This is called shortness of breath." In lung qì vacuity, the breathing function is debilitated and inhalation and exhalation is lessened with each breath. This manifests in debilitated breathing, dysphonia, and consequently in shortage of qì.

The chapter, "The Various Symptoms of Diseases of the Five Viscera and Six Bowels; Symptoms of Lung Disease" in the *Zhū Bìng Yuán Hòu Lùn* ("The Origin and Indicators of Disease") explains: "Insufficiency of lung qì results in shortage of qì and inability to breathe, deafness, and dry throat. All these indicate vacuity of lung qì." The chapter, "Shortage of Qì" in the *Zá Bìng Yuán Liú Xī Zhú* ("Incisive Light on the Source of Miscellaneous Disease") also explains:

> "The lung stores qì. Insufficiency of the lung results in faint breathing and shortage of qì… Vacuity of the lung results in qì having nowhere to be sorted and being unable to fill the qì storehouse. What is called shortage of qì is just like saying that there is not much to spare and that qì is vacuous and timid. It is not the same as the lack of continuous breathing that shortness of breath refers to."

This quote fully explains the pathomechanism by which lung qì vacuity and weakness can lead to numerous types of respiratory weaknesses.

This condition is treated by supplementing and boosting lung qì. The recommended formula is *bǔ fèi tāng* (Lung-Supplementing Decoction) from the *Yǒng Lèi Líng Fāng* ("Previously Published Formulas for the Benefit of All Posterity") with additions.

Bǔ Fèi Tāng 补肺汤 (Lung-Supplementing Decoction)
rén shēn 人参 (Ginseng Radix, ginseng)
huáng qí 黄耆 (Astragali Radix, astragalus)
shú dì huáng 熟地黄 (Rehmanniae Radix Praeparata, cooked rehmannia)
wǔ wèi zǐ 五味子 (Schisandrae Fructus, schisandra)
zǐ wǎn 紫菀 (Asteris Radix, aster)
sāng bái pí 桑白皮 (Mori Cortex, mulberry root bark)
Plus:
dōng chóng xià cǎo 冬虫夏草 (Cordyceps, cordyceps)
jié gěng 桔梗 (Platycodonis Radix, platycodon)

An alternative choice is *sì jūn zǐ tāng* (Four Gentlemen Decoction) from the *Tài Píng Huì Mín Hé Jì Jú Fāng* ("Tài-Píng Imperial Grace Pharmacy Formulas") with additions.

Sì Jūn Zǐ Tāng 四君子汤 (Four Gentlemen Decoction)
rén shēn 人参 (Ginseng Radix, ginseng)
bái zhú 白术 (Atractylodis Macrocephalae Rhizoma, white atractylodes)
fú líng 茯苓 (Poria, poria)
gān cǎo 甘草 (Glycyrrhizae Radix, licorice)
Plus:
huáng qí 黄耆 (Astragali Radix, astragalus)
bái guǒ 白果 (Ginkgo Semen, ginkgo)
wǔ wèi zǐ 五味子 (Schisandrae Fructus, schisandra)
yīng sù qiào (ké) 罂粟壳 (Papaveris Pericarpium, poppy husk)

呼吸无力

肺主气，司呼吸，吐故纳新，进行气体交换。各种原因损伤肺气，脏腑功能活动减弱，呼吸运动乏力，可引起一系列肺气虚弱的表现。肺气虚无力向上宣通鼻窍，可致鼻塞不通、嗅觉不灵。是因肺气通于鼻，肺和则能知香嗅。如果"肺气虚，则鼻塞不利"（《灵枢•本神篇》）。若肺气虚，不能推动肺叶收缩、舒张，宣发无能，肃降无权，肺气逆而上行，则出现咳逆流涕、咳喘无力、声低气怯、失音、动则尤甚等症。如《中藏经•论肺脏虚实寒热生死逆顺脉证》说："虚则力乏喘促，右胁胀，语言气短者是也。"若肺气虚，呼吸无力，每次呼出吸入之气减少，为满足全身供气的需要，呼吸频率被迫加快，病人感到不能报息，出现呼吸困难，名曰短气。正如《明医指掌•喘证》所云："若肺气太虚，气不能布息，呼吸不相接续，出多入少，名曰短气。"若肺气虚，呼吸功能衰弱，每次出入气息减少，表现为气息微弱、发音困难，则为少气。如《诸病源候论•五脏六腑病诸候•肺病候》说："肺气不足，则少气不能息，耳聋咽干，是为肺气之虚也。"《杂病源流犀烛•少气》也说："肺藏气，肺不足则息微少气，…肺虚则气无由藏，又不克充气之府。曰少气者，犹言所剩无多，虚虚怯怯，非如短气之不相接续也。"充分说明，肺气虚弱，可引起多种呼吸功能减弱的病机。治宜补益肺气。方选《永类钤方》补肺汤（黄芪、人参、熟地、五味子、紫菀、桑白皮）加虫草、桔梗。或选《和剂局方》四君子汤（人参、白术、茯苓、甘草）加黄芪、白果、五味、罂粟壳。

Literature Review of Forceless Breathing

📖 *Zhū Bìng Yuán Hòu Lùn* ("The Origin and Indicators of Disease"), "Lung Disease; Shortness of Breath"

> "Lung vacuity results in shortage and insufficiency of qì and also causes shortness of breath. Consequently, such a person presents with faint breath and often with shortage of qì and insufficiency in breathing."

This quotation discusses the pathomechanism by which lung qì vacuity and shortage and insufficiency of qì lead to shallow, short, and hasty breathing.

📖 *Zhāng Shì Yī Tōng* ("Zhang's Clear View of Medicine"), "On the Various Types of Qì; Panting"

> "Shortage of qì refers to qì being scant and insufficient. The classic states that timidity and shortage of qì mean that the water ways are stopped and that the qì of the body is dissipated. It also says that when a person speaks in a faint voice, [stopping] and speaking again only after a long time,speech is faint and the person only speaks again at the end of the day, this is a sign of despoliated qì…This condition is treated with formulas like *dú shēn tāng* (Pure Ginseng Decoction), *shēng mài sǎn* (Pulse-Engendering Powder), *bǎo yuán tāng* (Origin-Preserving Decoction), and *yì gōng sǎn* (Special Achievement Powder)."

The lung governs qì, and the pitch and strength of the voice is closely related to the exuberance and debilitation of lung qì. When lung qì is vacuous, inhalation and exhalation of breath are weakened. As a consequence, the sound of the voice is faint, low, and encumbered.

📖 *Tài Píng Shèng Huì Fāng* ("The Great Peace Sagacious Benevolence Formulary"), "Various Formulas for Treating Lung Qì Insufficiency"

> "The essence of the viscera and bowels all pours upward into the lung. The lung governs qì, which constitutes defense, flows into all the yáng

> channels, and luxuriates the skin and body hair. Insufficiency of its qì results in shortness of breath in the chest and diaphragm, block in the throat, cough and counterflow with snivel and spittle, cold that begins in the back, a sensation like holding snow in the mouth, loss of voice during speaking, and withered skin and body hair. All of these indicate insufficiency of lung qì."

This quotation discusses the pathomechanism by which lung qì vacuity, debilitated breathing, and impaired diffusion and depurative downbearing result in cough with counterflow and shortness of breath, coolness in the mouth and loss of voice, and dry skin and body hair.

文献评述

《诸病源候论•肺病候•短气候》曰:“肺虚则气少不足， 亦令短气， 则其人气微， 常如少气不足以呼吸。”论述肺气虚， 气少不足， 而致呼吸表浅短促的病机。

《张氏医通•诸气门•喘》曰:“少气者， 气少不足以言也。经曰: 怯然少气者， 是水道不行， 形气消索也。又云: 言而微， 终日乃复言者， 此夺气也。…其治法不离独参汤、生脉散、保元汤、异功散之类。”肺主气， 声音的高低强弱与肺气的盛衰有着密切的关系。肺气虚， 则呼吸的气息减弱， 故说话语声低微、困难。

《太平圣惠方•治肺气不足诸方》曰:“夫脏腑之精， 皆上注于肺。肺主于气， 气为卫， 流注于诸阳之经， 荣华于皮毛。若其气不足， 则胸膈短气， 咽中闭塞， 咳逆涕唾， 寒从背起， 口中如含霜雪， 语言失声， 皮毛萎瘁， 皆肺气不足之候也。”论述肺气虚， 呼吸功能衰退， 宣发肃降乏力， 引起咳逆短气， 口冷失声， 皮毛枯萎的病机。

Summary of Forceless Breathing

1. Lack of Strength in Perfusing the Orifices of the Lung
   Nasal congestion, poor sense of smell.
2. Lung Qì Lacking Strength for Depurative Downbearing
   Cough and counterflow with snivel, cough with panting and lack of strength, low voice and qì timidity, loss of voice.
3. Shallow and Accelerated Breathing
   Encumbered breathing, which is called shortness of breath.
4. Inhalation and Exhalation Lessened with Each Breath
   Faint breathing, shortage of qì with difficulty speaking.

呼吸无力
无力宣通肺窍——鼻塞不通，嗅觉不灵。 无力肃降肺气——咳逆流涕、咳喘无力， 声低气怯，失音。 呼吸表浅频率加快——呼吸困难，名曰短气。 每次出入气息减少——气息微弱，少气难言。

4.2 Insecurity of External Defense

The lung governs the skin and body hair. When lung qì is vacuous, it is unable to effuse defense qì. As a result, defense yáng is unable to spread into the skin, safeguarding lacks strength, the interstices of the flesh are loosened, and the fluids are discharged outward. At the same time, external evil is able to exploit the vacuity, enter the body, and damage defense qì, resulting in construction and defense disorders. This manifests in symptoms like spontaneous sweating, aversion to wind, susceptibility to the common cold, a pale tongue with thin tongue fur, and a vacuous and forceless pulse.

The "Schema of Miscellaneous Patterns; Sweating" in the *Jǐng Yuè Quán Shū* ("Jǐng-Yuè's Complete Compendium") states: "Spontaneous sweating is ascribed to yáng vacuity and insecurity of the interstices. It is a function of defense qì. People use defense qì to secure the exterior. Insecurity of defense qì results in exterior vacuity and spontaneous sweating, as a result of which the fluids are discharged." The reference to yáng vacuity in this source does not mean that yáng qì fails to warm, but that the lung's qì is vacuous and unable to diffuse defense qì. The chapter, "Lung Vacuity Cough" in the *Bù Jū Jí* ("The Variability Collection") also explains:

> "Lung vacuity means that the lung itself lacks qì and therefore becomes vacuous. If it is vacuous, the interstices do not close tightly, and as a result the person is externally averse to wind without wind being present, and averse to cold without cold being present."

This source further illustrates the pathomechanism by which lung vacuity and insecurity of external defense cause a variety of manifestations.

This condition is treated by supplementing and boosting lung qì, and by securing the exterior and checking sweating. The recommended formula is *yù píng fēng sǎn* (Jade Wind-Barrier Powder) from the *Dān Xī Xīn Fǎ* ("Dān Xī's Heart-Approach") with additions.

Yù Píng Fēng Săn 玉屏风散 (Jade Wind-Barrier Powder)
huáng qí 黄耆 (Astragali Radix, astragalus)
bái zhú 白朮 (Atractylodis Macrocephalae Rhizoma, white atractylodes)
fáng fēng 防风 (Saposhnikoviae Radix, saposhnikovia)
Plus:
fú xiăo mài 浮小麦 (Tritici Fructus Levis, light wheat)
duàn lóng gŭ 煅龙骨 (Mastodi Ossis Fossilia Calcinata, calcined dragon bone)
má huáng gēn 麻黄根 (Ephedrae Radix, ephedra root)
nuò dào gēn xū 糯稻根 (Oryzae Glutinosae Radix, glutinous rice root)

卫外不固

肺主皮毛， 肺气虚， 不能宣发卫气， 卫阳不能布敷肌表， 固护无力， 肌腠疏松， 津液外泄， 同时外邪也会乘虚而入， 损伤卫气， 导致营卫失调。表现为自汗、恶风、易于感冒、舌淡苔薄， 脉虚无力等症。如《景岳全书•杂证谟•汗证》云: "自汗者属阳虚， 腠理不固， 卫气之所司也。人以卫气固其表， 卫气不固， 则表虚自汗， 而津液为之发泄也。" 这里的阳虚， 不指阳气失于温煦， 而是指肺的气虚不能宣发卫气。《不居集•肺虚咳嗽》又说: "肺虚者， 肺家无气自虚也。惟其自虚， 则腠理不密， 故外则无风而畏风， 外则无寒而恶寒。" 则进一步阐明肺虚卫外不固而引起各种表现的机理。治宜补益肺气， 固表止汗。方选《丹溪心法》玉屏风散（黄芪、白术、防风）加浮小麦、煅龙牡、麻黄根、糯稻根。

Literature Review of Insecurity of External Defense

🕮 *Biàn Zhèng Lù* ("Records on Pattern Differentiation"), "Sweating Pattern"

> "After severe illness, the lung will invariably be injured first. If the lung first lacks the power to govern itself, how can it counter the insecurity of its qì? Given the fact that sweat is transformed qì, an insecurity of qì causes sweat to follow qì and be discharged, resulting in dripping sweat all over the body."

This quotation describes the pathomechanism by which damage to lung qì after disease causes lung qì vacuity and insecurity of external defense, resulting in spontaneous persistent sweating.

🕮 *Bìng Jī Huì Lùn* ("Collected Discussions on Pathomechanisms"), "Section on Spontaneous Sweating and Night Sweating"

> "In spontaneous sweating, the disease is located in the lung. Defense qì is insecure, the interstices are not tightly closed, and sweat follows qì to be dissipated."

This quotation discusses the pathomechanism by which lung qì vacuity, insecurity of external defense, and poorly closed interstices lead to spontaneous sweating.

📖 *Gŭ Jīn Yī Jiàn* ("Mirror of Medicine Ancient and Modern"), "Spontaneous Sweating and Night Sweating"

> "Constant spontaneous sweating that is not caused by disease, and profuse sweating after disease, are ascribed to exterior vacuity and insecurity of defense qì, and to construction-blood leaking out. They should be treated with *huáng qí jiàn zhōng tāng* (Astragalus Center-Fortifying Decoction) supplemented with *fú mài jiān* (Dry Fried Tritici Fructus levis), or with *huáng qí liù yī tāng* (Astragalus Six-To-One Decoction) or *yù píng fēng săn* (Jade Wind-Barrier Powder)."

Exterior vacuity and insecurity of external defense are caused by lung qì vacuity and impaired external defense, which causes discharge of construction-blood and spontaneous sweating. The formulas for *huáng qí jiàn zhōng tāng* (Astragalus Center-Fortifying Decoction) and *yù píng fēng săn* (Jade Wind-Barrier Powder) are perfect for supplementing lung qì and securing the defensive exterior.

文献评述

《辨证录•汗证门》曰: "大病之后， 必先损其肺， 肺先无自主之权， 安能禁其气之不固哉。气不固， 而汗乃气之所化， 汗随气泄， 遍体出汗淋漓。" 论述病后伤肺气， 肺气虚而卫外不固， 自汗不止的病机。

《病机汇论•自汗盗汗门》曰: "自汗者， 其病在肺， 卫气不固， 腠理不密， 而汗随气散也。" 论述肺气虚， 卫外不固， 腠理失密， 引起自汗的病机。

《古今医鉴•自汗盗汗》曰: "其无病而汗常自出， 与病后多汗， 皆属表虚卫气不固， 荣血泄漏， 宜黄芪建中汤加浮麦煎， 黄芪六一汤或玉屏风散。" 表虚卫外不固， 是因肺气虚卫外失职， 才使营血外泄而为自汗， 所用黄芪建中汤、玉屏风散全是补肺气而固卫表的方剂。

Summary of Insecurity of External Defense
Insecurity of External Defense Profuse sweating, fear of wind, susceptibility to the common cold.
卫外不固
自汗， 畏风， 易于感冒。

4.3 Stoppage of the Fluids

The lung is the upper source of water. Stoppage of the fluids can occur in two different pathomechanisms: First, an invasion of evil qì or retention of pathologic substances can cause lung block due to evil repletion. As a result, the lung fails to diffuse and depurate and becomes unable to regulate the waterways, causing stoppage of the fluids. As a second alternative, a weakness of lung qì can prevent it from carrying out diffusion and depuration. Consequently, it lacks strength to propel the fluids, the waterways are stopped, and fluids collect. This can also cause phlegm-rheum. Normally, this condition manifests in cough and vomiting of profuse thin clear white phlegm-drool.

The chapter, "Phlegm-Rheum" in the *Yī Mén Fǎ Lǜ* ("Axioms of Medicine") explains: "The lung governs qì, moves construction and defense, and distributes the fluids. When qì congeals, humor gathers and transmutes into foamy drool." While congealing qì can be caused by cold, it can also be due to qì vacuity causing forceless promotion of movement. When lung qì is vacuous, qì fails to transform liquid, and liquid fails to bear upward. This results in dryness in the mouth and thirst with desire to drink water.

This is exactly what the following quotation references: "When the lung fails to regulate, ancestral qì is not distributed, causing shortness of breath. When qì is not distributed, liquid is not transformed, causing thirst with dryness in the diaphragm." These types of dryness and thirst conditions are extremely easy to mistake for heat signs and must be noted with special attention in clinic.

When lung qì is vacuous and therefore unable to diffuse, to propel, and to transform liquid, liquid can flood and collect in the head and face. This can lead to cough with puffy swelling of the face and eyes. As the "Treatise on Cough" in the *Tài Píng Shèng Huì Fāng* ("The Great Peace Sagacious Benevolence Formulary") states:

> "The lung governs qì and is reflected in the skin and body hair. In its movement, qì encircles the viscera and bowels and pours into the channels and network vessels. When a weakness of lung qì is exploited by lung evil, the skin is blocked, which causes qì to congest internally. Together with humor, it is unable to diffuse and consequently spills into the skin. This causes cough with puffy swelling of the face and eyes."

This quotation explains how lung qì vacuity, weak qì, and obstruction of liquid can lead to puffy swelling.

This condition is treated by supplementing and boosting lung qì, and by fortifying the spleen and transforming phlegm. The recommended formula is *liù jūn zǐ tāng* (Six Gentlemen Decoction) from the *Fù Rén Liáng Fāng* ("Good Remedies for Women") with additions.

Liù Jūn Zǐ Tāng 六君子汤 (Six Gentlemen Decoction)
rén shēn 人参 (Ginseng Radix, ginseng)
fú líng 茯苓 (Poria, poria)
bái zhú 白朮 (Atractylodis Macrocephalae Rhizoma, white atractylodes)
bàn xià 半夏 (Pinelliae Rhizoma, pinellia)
chén pí 陈皮 (Citri Reticulatae Pericarpium, tangerine peel)
gān cǎo 甘草 (Glycyrrhizae Radix, licorice)
Plus:
huáng qí 黄耆 (Astragali Radix, astragalus)
zǐ wǎn 紫菀 (Asteris Radix, aster)
kuǎn dōng huā 款冬花 (Farfarae Flos, coltsfoot)

津液不行

肺为水之上源，除受邪气侵袭或病理产物停留，邪实肺闭，肺失宣肃，不能通调水道而致津液不行外，当其肺气虚弱，不行宣肃之职，无力推动津液运行，水道不通，津液停滞，亦可化生痰饮。常见咳嗽，呕吐痰涎，色白清稀量多等症。正如《医门法律•痰饮》所说: “肺主气，行营卫，布津液，气凝则液聚，变成涎沫。”气凝虽可由寒凝引起，但亦包括因气虚无力推动所致。若肺气虚，气不化津，津不上承，则为口中干燥、渴欲饮水。此乃“肺之治节不行，宗气不布，故短气；气不布则津亦不化，故膈燥而渴”（《医门法律•痰饮脉论》）。此类燥渴症，极易误辨为热象，临床尤当注意。若肺气虚，不得宣泄，失于推动，气不化津，水津泛溢，停留头面，可引起咳嗽，面目浮肿。如《太平圣惠方•咳嗽论》云: “夫肺主于气，候于皮毛，而气之行，循环脏腑，流注经络，若肺气虚弱，肺邪所乘，则肌肤否塞，使气内壅，与液相并，不得宣泄，致溢皮肤，故令咳嗽而面目浮肿。”说明肺气虚，气弱津阻，可致浮肿。治宜补益肺气，健脾化痰。方选《妇人良方》六君子汤（人参、茯苓、白术、半夏、陈皮、甘草）加黄芪、紫菀、冬花。

Literature Review of Stoppage of the Fluids

📖 *Qiān Jīn Yào Fāng* (“A Thousand Gold Pieces Prescriptions”), “Lung Vacuity and Repletion; Lung Vacuity Cold”

“Insufficiency of lung qì manifests in cough, counterflow, and shortness of breath; in cold that arises from the back and a sensation in the mouth

> as if holding snow there; in loss of voice and thirst, and in dryness at the root of the tongue."

This quotation describes how lung qì vacuity prevents qì from transforming liquid, and liquid from bearing upward, which causes cold sensation in the mouth, dryness, and thirst.

🕮 *Lín Zhèng Zhǐ Nán Yī Àn* ("A Clinical Guide with Case Histories"), "Phlegm-Rheum" Zōu Zī-Jiǔ's commentary

> "Summing up the action of phlegm-rheum, it is invariably caused by depletion of original qì and resulting yīn exuberance with yáng debilitation. These cause the fluids to congeal and stagnate instead of being distributed, and to collect inside the chest, so that the clearness of water is completely transformed into turbidity. When water causes yīn to accumulate, rheum results; when rheum causes yáng to congeal, phlegm results."

This quotation illustrates how the formation of phlegm-rheum is caused by depletion of original qì, by qì failing to transform liquid, and by fluids congealing and collecting inside the chest.

文献评述

《千金要方•肺虚实•肺虚冷》曰:“肺气不足，咳逆气短，寒从背起，口中如含霜雪，语无音声而渴，舌本干燥。”论述肺气虚，气不化津，津不上承，可致口中冷，干燥而渴。

《临证指南医案•痰饮》邹滋九按语:“总之痰饮之作，必由元气亏乏，及阴盛阳衰而起，以致津液凝滞，不能输布，留于胸中，水之清者悉变为浊，水积阴则为饮，饮凝阳则为痰。”阐明痰饮形成的病机是由元气亏损，气不化津，津液凝滞，停于胸中所致。

Summary of Stoppage of the Fluids
1. Weak Qì and Collecting Liquid Cough, vomiting of profuse amounts of clear white thin phlegm-drool.
2. Qì Failing to Move Liquid Dryness inside the mouth, thirst with desire to drink water.
3. Qì Failing to Move Water Cough, puffy swelling of the face and eyes.

津液不行
气弱津停——咳嗽，呕吐痰涎，色白清稀量多。
气不行津——口中干燥，渴欲饮水。
气不行水——咳嗽，面目浮肿。

4.4 Failure of the Upper Body to Control the Lower Body

The urinary bladder has the function of storing and eliminating urine; it is related to the kidney's action of steaming qì transformation; and in addition, it is subject to control by lung qì. If lung qì is weak and unable to govern depurative downbearing, this affects qì transformation in the bladder by impairing bladder retention. The resulting condition in which the bladder opens easily but closes with difficulty manifests in symptoms like enuresis and incontinence.

The chapter, "Discussing the Pulses and Patterns of Vacuity and Repletion, Cold and Heat, Life and Death, and Favorable and Unfavorable Shifts in the Viscera and Bowels" in the *Zhōng Zàng Jīng* ("Central Treasury Canon") stated: "Cough with enuresis means upper body vacuity and inability to control the lower body." Huà Tuó was the first to mention the pathomechanism of upper body failing to control the lower body. He pointed out that enuresis after cough allowed one to know that vacuity in the upper body was lung qì vacuity.

In the chapter, "Creating Formulas by Differentiating the Channels According to the Disease" in the *Pí Wèi Lùn* ("On the Spleen and Stomach") Lǐ Dōng-Yuán explained, "Enuresis means lung qì vacuity," thereby providing further evidence for this pathomechanism.

The chapter, "The Internal Organs" in the *Yī Xué Rù Mén* ("The Gateway to Medicine") elaborated this further: "Vacuity of lung qì results in breathing with shortage of qì, insufficient respiration, and frequent urination or enuresis." By explicating treating disease in the lower body through the upper body, this text laid the theoretical foundation for the method of treating enuresis by supplementing the lung.

This condition is treated by supplementing and boosting lung qì. The recommended formula is *bǎo yuán tāng* (Origin-Preserving Decoction), which uses sweet and warming medicinals to supplement and boost lung qì, and by making lung qì effulgent, enable the upper body to control the lower body, so that urinary emission is controlled on its own.

Bǎo Yuán Tāng 保元汤 (Origin-Preserving Decoction)
huáng qí 黄芪 (Astragali Radix, astragalus)
rén shēn 人参 (Ginseng Radix, ginseng)
ròu guì 肉桂 (Cinnamomi Cortex, cinnamon bark)
gān cǎo 甘草 (Glycyrrhizae Radix, licorice)

Enuresis that is due to bladder retention failure caused by taxation damage from excessive anxiety and thought and resultant vacuity of lung and spleen qì must be treated by supplementing the lung and fortifying the spleen. The recommended formula is *bǔ zhōng yì qì tāng* (Center-Supplementing Qì-Boosting Decoction) with additions.

Bǔ Zhōng Yì Qì Tāng 补中益气汤 (Center-Supplementing Qì-Boosting Decoction)
huáng qí 黄耆 (Astragali Radix, astragalus)
zhì gān cǎo (炙甘草 Glycyrrhizae Radix Praeparata, mix-fried licorice)
rén shēn 人参 (Ginseng Radix, ginseng)
bái zhú 白朮 (Atractylodis Macrocephalae Rhizoma, white atractylodes)
dāng guī 当归 (Angelicae Sinensis Radix, Chinese angelica)
chén pí 陈皮 (Citri Reticulatae Pericarpium, tangerine peel)
shēng má 升麻 (Cimicifugae Rhizoma, cimicifuga)
chái hú 柴胡 (Bupleuri Radix, bupleurum)
Plus:
mǔ lì 牡蛎 (Ostreae Concha, oyster shell)
wǔ wèi zǐ 五味子 (Schisandrae Fructus, schisandra)

The lung and the large intestine stand in exterior-interior relationship. Depurative downbearing by lung qì can cause the fluids to percolate down into the large intestine. At the same time, the lung also assists the large intestine in its conveyance function and safeguards the smooth elimination of stool, by moistening and promoting uninhibited flow. If lung qì is insufficient, depurative downbearing is impaired, and the fluids are unable to percolate downward. Lung qì fails to propel movement and large intestinal conveyance is impaired, which retards intestinal peristalsis. This can lead to vacuity constipation, and to forceless defecation.

In the *Yī Guàn* ("Thorough Knowledge of Medicine"), "Constipation," Zhào Xiàn advocated the use of *rén shēn* (Ginseng Radix) and *huáng qí* (Astragali Radix) in the treatment of constipation due to qì vacuity and shortage of fluids in the elderly. He explained this recommendation in the following fashion: "This condition is caused by qì being vacuous and therefore unable to propel and deliver, and by yīn being vacuous and therefore unable to moisten." While he did not yet directly mention lung qì vacuity as the cause, he treated it with *rén shēn* (Ginseng Radix) and *huáng qí* (Astragali Radix), both of which effect the supplementation and boosting of lung qì. By supplementing lung qì, empowering depurative downbearing, and strengthening intestinal movement, thus spontaneously freeing the stool, he was able to treat constipation. Thus, he provided indirect proof for the pathomechanism by which lung qì vacuity can cause constipation.

This condition is treated by supplementing the lung and boosting qì, and by moistening the intestines and freeing the stool. The recommended formula is *wēi líng xiān wán* (Clematis Pill) from the *Shì Yī Dé Xiào Fāng* ("Effective Formula From a Family Tradition") with additions.

Wēi Líng Xiān Wán 威灵仙丸 (Clematis Pill)
huáng qí 黄耆 (Astragali Radix, astragalus)
zhǐ shí 枳实 (Aurantii Fructus Immaturus, unripe bitter orange)
wēi líng xiān 威灵仙 (Clematidis Radix, clematis)
Plus:
rén shēn 人参 (Ginseng Radix, ginseng)
bái zhú 白朮 (Atractylodis Macrocephalae Rhizoma, white atractylodes)
yì mǔ cǎo 益母草 (Leonuri Herba, leonurus)

Alternatively, *huáng qí tāng* (Astragalus Decoction) from the *Jīn Guì Yì* ("The Wings of the Golden Coffer") with additions is used.

Huáng Qí Tāng 黄耆汤 (Astragalus Decoction)
huáng qí 黄耆 (Astragali Radix, astragalus)
chén pí 陈皮 (Citri Reticulatae Pericarpium, tangerine peel)
huǒ má rén 火麻仁 (Cannabis Fructus, cannabis fruit)
bái zhú 白朮 (Atractylodis Macrocephalae Rhizoma, white atractylodes)
Plus:
shēng má 升麻 (Cimicifugae Rhizoma, cimicifuga)
jié gěng 桔梗 (Platycodonis Radix, platycodon)
rén shēn 人参 (Ginseng Radix, ginseng)

上不制下

膀胱有贮尿、排尿的功能，除与肾的蒸腾气化有关外，还受到肺气的制约。若肺气虚弱，不能主司肃降，影响膀胱气化，失却对膀胱的制约，膀胱处于易开难合的状态，则形成小便遗失，或失禁等症。《中藏经•论脏腑虚实寒热生死逆顺脉证》曰："咳而遗溺者，上虚不能制下也。”华佗最早提出上不制下的病机，从咳而引起遗尿，可知上虚系指肺气虚。李东垣《脾胃论•分经随病制方》说:“小便遗失者，肺气虚也。”对此病机作了进一步肯定。《医学入门•脏腑》亦补充说:“肺之气，虚则呼吸少气，不足以息，小便频数或遗。”为下病上治，治疗遗尿病用补肺法的创立奠定了理论基础。治宜补益肺气，方选保元汤（黄芪、人参、桂心、甘草），以甘温药补益肺气，肺气旺，上能制下，小便遗失自然得到控制。若劳伤忧思过度，肺脾气虚，不能约束膀胱，而为小便遗溺，又当补肺健脾，用补中益气汤加牡蛎、五味子治疗。

肺与大肠相表里，肺气肃降，可使津液下渗大肠。同时亦协助大肠传导功能，保证大便顺利排泄，润泽通畅。如果肺气不足，失于肃降，津液不能下渗，肺气失于推动，大肠传导失职，肠的蠕动减慢，可致大便虚秘，无力排泄。赵献可在治疗老年人气虚、津液衰少，而致便秘，主张加人参、黄芪，并阐述病机说:“此因气虚不能推送，阴虚不能濡润耳”（《医贯•大便不通》）。虽未确认为肺气虚所致，但在治疗时使用中药人参、黄芪，均有补益肺气的作用，肺气得补，肃降有权，运肠有力，便自通畅，可免受便秘之苦，又间接反证肺气虚可致便秘的病机。治宜补肺益气，润肠通便。方选《世医得效方》威灵仙丸（黄芪、枳实、威灵仙）加人参、白术、益母草。亦可用《金匮翼》黄芪汤（黄芪、陈皮、麻仁、白密）加升麻、桔梗、人参。

Literature Review of Failure of the Upper Body to Control the Lower Body

🕮 *Jīn Guì Yì* (“The Wings of the Golden Coffer”), “Urinary Incontinence”

> “Vacuity of qì in the lung and spleen, inability to retain the waterways, and resultant incontinence is what the *Jīn Guì Yào Lüe* (“Essential Prescriptions of the Golden Coffer”) refers to as upper body vacuity and inability to control the lower body.”

This quotation describes precisely how lung qì vacuity and inability to carry out depuration can impair bladder retention and cause spontaneous urinary emission.

🕮 *Zhèng Yīn Mài Zhì* (“Pathoconditions: Causes, Pulses, and Treatments”), “Treatise on Constipation”

> “If original qì is insufficient and lung qì is unable to reach the lower body, the large intestine is unable to carry out conveyance and the stool is bound.” “The pulse of qì constipation and bound stool: Fine and faint at the

> right inch position, indicating insufficiency of lung qì." "The treatment of qì constipation and bound stool: For lung vacuity and inability to reach the lower body, use *shēng mài sǎn* (Pulse-Engendering Powder) in combination with *shēn jú jiān* (Fried Ginseng and Tangerine Peel)."

This quotation discusses not only how lung qì vacuity and impaired depurative downbearing and promotion of movement by qì can lead to constipation, but it also describes the pulse manifestation and treatment method.

文献评述

《金匮翼•小便不禁》曰: "肺脾气虚，不能约束水道而病为不禁者，<金匮>所谓上虚不能制下者也。" 明确论述肺气虚，不行清肃之令，可致膀胱不约而小便自遗。

《症因脉治•大便秘结论》曰 "若元气不足，肺气不能下达，则大肠不得传道之令，而大便亦结矣。" "气秘便结之脉: 右寸细微，肺气不足。" "气秘便结之治: 肺虚不能下达，生脉散合参橘煎。" 不仅论述肺气虚，气失肃降推动无力，可致大便秘结，而且描述其脉象及治法。

Summary of Failure of the Upper Body to Control the Lower Body
1. Lung Vacuity and Bladder Retention Failure Enuresis or incontinence. 2. Lung Vacuity and Forceless Promotion of Movement Vacuity constipation, forceless defecation.

上不制下
肺虚膀胱失制——小便遗失，或失禁。 肺虚推动无力——大便虚秘，无力排泄。

4.5 Debilitation of Ancestral Qì

> "The lung governs ancestral qì and moves it around the whole body (*Chóng Dìng Tōng Sú Shāng Hán Lùn* ("Revised Popular On Cold Damage"), "Vacuity and Repletion of Qì and Blood; Qì Vacuity Patterns")."

When lung qì is insufficient, it is unable to form ancestral qì. This can easily lead to debilitation and shortage of ancestral qì. Ancestral qì has the functions of moving breath in the respiratory tract, governing respiration, and moving qì and blood through the heart vessel. Debilitation of ancestral qì can induce three different pathomechanisms:

宗气衰少

"肺主宗气而运行周身"（《重订通俗伤寒论•气血虚实•气虚证》），肺气不足，不能化生宗气，易致宗气衰少。宗气有行息道主呼吸和贯心脉行气血的作用，宗气衰少，其病机有三:

4.5.1 Dysphonia

Zhāng Jǐng-Yuè explained: "The voice emits sound because of qì, and insufficiency of qì causes light and timid speech and inability to make sound (*Lèi Jīng* ("The Classified Canon"), "Categories of Channels and Network Vessels; The Four Seas of Humans")." When insufficiency of lung qì has debilitated ancestral qì, it is unable to rouse qì to flow and surge up into the throat. Consequently, the production of sound lacks strength. This manifests in symptoms such as low voice and qì timidity, shortage of qì and laziness to speak, breathing with weak qì, and cough, panting, and a low voice.

The "Treatise on Seas" in the *Líng Shū* ("The Magic Pivot") states: "Insufficiency in the sea of qì results in qì being insufficient for speaking." The sea of qì is the center of the chest; what is stored inside the chest is ancestral qì. Thus, insufficiency in the sea of qì refers to debilitation of ancestral qì, which causes qì shortage and difficulty in sustaining the production of sound and speaking. The *Lèi Jīng* ("The Classified Canon"), "Categories of Diseases; Death from Loss of Guard and Loss of Strength" explains: "Extreme qì vacuity causes the voice to be discontinuous and the lung to lose its ancestor." This quotation provides ample clarification for the pathomechanism by which lung qì vacuity and debilitation of ancestral qì lead to low voice and laziness to speak. Even more clearly, the chapter, "Treating Enduring Muteness by Supplementing Original Qì and Bringing About Spontaneous Opening" in the *Gǔ Jīn Yī Tǒng Dà Quán* ("The Complete Compendium of Medical Works, Ancient and Modern"); "Sound of the Voice" points out:

> "All enduring cough with muteness is related to insufficiency of original qì and to lung qì failing to enrich. It should be treated by supplementing qì, nourishing metal, and moistening dryness, to make the voice naturally resonant."

The recommended formula for dysphonia is *rén shēn píng bǔ tāng* (Ginseng Balanced Supplementation Decoction) from the same text, with the addition of *hē zǐ* (Chebulae Fructus). By treating the kidney, supplementing the lung, and boosting metal qì, this formula has the effect of supplementing the origin, boosting qì, and increasing the voice.

Rén Shēn Píng Bǔ Tāng 人参平补汤
(Ginseng Balanced Supplementation Decoction)

rén shēn 人参 (Ginseng Radix, ginseng)
wǔ wèi zǐ 五味子 (Schisandrae Fructus, schisandra)
dāng guī 当归 (Angelicae Sinensis Radix, Chinese angelica)
chuān xiōng 川芎 (Chuanxiong Rhizoma, chuanxiong)
bái sháo 白芍 (Paeoniae Radix Alba, white peony)
shú dì huáng 熟地黄 (Rehmanniae Radix Praeparata, cooked rehmannia)
tù sī zǐ 菟丝子 (Cuscutae Semen, cuscuta)
bǔ gǔ zhī 补骨脂 (Psoraleae Fructus, psoralea)
yì zhì rén 益智仁 (Alpiniae Oxyphyllae Fructus, alpinia)
hú lú bā 胡芦巴 (Trigonellae Semen, fenugreek)
bā jǐ tiān 巴戟天 (Morindae Officinalis Radix, morinda)
dù zhòng 杜仲 (Eucommiae Cortex, eucommia)
bái zhú 白朮 (Atractylodis Macrocephalae Rhizoma, white atractylodes)
jú hóng 橘红 (Citri Reticulatae Pericarpium Rubrum, red tangerine peel)
bàn xià qū 半夏曲 (Pinelliae Massa Fermentata, pinellia leaven)
shí chāng pú 石菖蒲 (Acori Tatarinowii Rhizoma, acorus)
gān cǎo 甘草 (Glycyrrhizae Radix, licorice)

Plus:
hē zǐ 诃子 (Chebulae Fructus, chebule)

发音困难

张景岳说："声由气发，气不足则语言轻怯，不能出声"（《类经•经络类•人之四海》）。肺气不足，宗气衰少，不能振奋气流，上冲咽喉，发声无力，则见声低气怯、少气懒言、呼吸气弱、咳喘声低等症。如《灵枢•海论篇》曰："气海不足，则气少不足以言。"胸中为气海，胸中所藏为宗气，气海不足，即言宗气虚衰，气少难以维持发音、说话。《类经•疾病类•失守失强者死》说："气虚之甚，故声不接续，肺脏失宗也。"充分阐明肺气虚，宗气衰少引起声低懒言的病机。《古今医统大全•声音门•治久病声哑宜补元气自开》更明确提出"凡病人久嗽声哑，乃是元气不足，肺气不滋，宜补气养金润燥，其声自亮。"处方宜选该书人参平补汤（人参、五味、当归、川芎、白芍、熟地、菟丝子、补骨脂、益智仁、芦巴、巴戟、杜仲、白术、橘红、半夏曲、石菖蒲、甘草）加柯子，治肾补肺益金气，而收补元益气增声之功。

4.5.2 Qì Failing to Moving Blood

The lung assembles the hundred vessels and governs management and regulating. Ancestral qì has the function of assisting the heart in moving blood by connecting with the heart vessel. When lung qì is vacuous, ancestral qì is debilitated and unable to promote the flow of blood. This manifests in two different pathomechanisms: In the first, vacuous lung qì lacks the strength to upbear, and ancestral qì is unable to move blood upward to luxuriate the face. This can result in symptoms like a pale white facial complexion and pale lips and tongue. In the second, ancestral qì that is vacuous and deficient is unable to assist the heart in moving blood. This causes qì vacuity with blood stasis, blood impediment in the heart vessel, and blood obstructing lung qì. It manifests in symptoms like heart palpitations and fearful throbbing, oppression and stifling pain in the chest, a dark purple facial complexion, and green-blue or purple lips and nails.

Both of these pathomechanisms are treated by supplementing qì, quickening blood, and freeing the impediment. The recommended formula is *bǔ yáng huán wǔ tāng* (Yáng-Supplementing Five-Returning Decoction) from the *Yī Lín Gǎi Cuò* ("Correction of Errors in Medical Classics") with the addition of *rén shēn* (Ginseng Radix) and *guì zhī* (Cinnamomi Ramulus).

Bǔ Yáng Huán Wǔ Tāng 补阳还五汤 (Yáng-Supplementing Five-Returning Decoction)
huáng qí 黄耆 (Astragali Radix, astragalus)
dāng guī 当归 (Angelicae Sinensis Radix, Chinese angelica)
chuān xiōng 川芎 (Chuanxiong Rhizoma, chuanxiong)
táo rén 桃仁 (Persicae Semen, peach kernel)
chì sháo 芍药 (Paeoniae Radix Rubra, red peony)
dì lóng 地龙 (Pheretima, earthworm)
Plus:
rén shēn 人参 (Ginseng Radix, ginseng)
guì zhī 桂枝 (Cinnamomi Ramulus, cinnamon twig)

气不行血

肺朝百脉，主治节，宗气有贯心脉助心行血的作用。肺气虚，宗气衰，不能推动血行，有两方面的病机。一是肺气虚，无力上升，宗气不能运血上荣于面，可见面色淡白、唇舌色淡诸症。二是宗气虚少，不能助心行血，气虚血瘀，血痹心脉，血阻肺气，可见心悸怔忡、胸闷憋痛、面色紫暗、唇甲青紫等症。治宜补气活血通痹。方选《医林改错》补阳还五汤（黄芪、归尾、川芎、桃仁、赤芍、地龙）加人参、桂枝。

4.5.3 Downward Fall of Great Qì

Great qì is directly tied to the qì inside the lung, and is in fact identical with ancestral qi. As Yù Jiā-Yán explained, "What is sometimes referred to as great qì is just another name for ancestral qì. Ancestral expresses veneration and ancestry." Zhāng Xī-Chún further pointed out:

> "The true reason for the lung's ability to breathe is found in the great qì inside the lung… Moreover, this qì is able to sustain the entire body and arouse the essence-spirit, engage the heart and thought in mental activities, and activate the five viscera and structure of the body. All of these rely on it."

When lung qì is effulgent, ancestral qì is plentiful and the great qì within the lung bears upward and downward with facility, resulting in normal breathing and coordinated organ functions. But when lung qì is weak, ancestral qì is debilitated and the great qì inside the chest does not move. Great qì falling downward instead of rising up can lead to symptoms like shortness of breath, labored exhalation, faint breathing, fatigue and lack of strength in the entire body, devitalized essence-spirit, slowness of thought, and at critical times, sudden stopped breathing.

The "Treatise on Great Qì" in the *Yī Mén Fǎ Lǜ* ("Axioms of Medicine") explains thusly:

> "As great qì is debilitated, the breathing feels inhibited. Moreover, the limbs are sore and lazy and the essence-spirit clouded and fretting, which causes a sudden reduction in mental capabilities. If the qì is not only vacuous, but falls downward, possibly too severely, such a person experiences sudden stopped breathing and clouding loss of consciousness."

Downward fall of great qì manifests most prominently in the pathomechanical trends of lung qì vacuity, failure of lung qì to rise, and in severe cases, downward desertion.

Downward fall of great qì is treated by boosting qì and upbearing the fall. The recommended formula is *shēng xiàn tāng* (Fall-Upbearing Decoction) from the *Yī Xué Zhōng Zhōng Cān Xī Lù* ("Records of Chinese Medicine with Reference to Western Medicine") with additions.

Shēng Xiàn Tāng 升陷汤 (Fall-Upbearing Decoction)
huáng qí 黄耆 (Astragali Radix, astragalus)
chái hú 柴胡 (Bupleuri Radix, bupleurum)
shēng má 升麻 (Cimicifugae Rhizoma, cimicifuga)
jié gěng 桔梗 (Platycodonis Radix, platycodon)
Plus:
rén shēn 人参 (Ginseng Radix, ginseng)
shān zhū yú 山茱萸 (Corni Fructus, cornus)

大气下陷

大气系指胸中之气，大气即是宗气。正如喻嘉言所说："或谓大气即宗气之别名，宗者，尊也、祖也"（《医门法律•大气论》）。张锡纯进一步指出："肺之所以能呼吸者，实赖胸中之大气。…而此气，且能撑持全身，振作精神，以及心思脑力、官骸动作，莫不赖乎此气"（《医学衷中参西录•升陷汤》）。肺气旺盛，宗气充足，胸中大气升降自如，则呼吸正常，脏腑功能协调。肺气虚弱，宗气衰少，胸中大气不转，大气不升，反而下陷，可致短气、呼出困难、气息微弱、全身倦怠乏力、精神不振、思维迟钝等症，严重时可见呼吸顿停。《医门法律•大气论》说："大气一衰，呼吸即觉不利，而且肢体酸懒，精神昏愦，脑力心思，为之顿减。若其气虚而且陷，或下陷过甚，其人则呼吸顿停，昏然罔觉。"大气下陷，着重表现肺气虚弱，肺气不升，甚至下脱的病机趋势。治宜益气升陷。方选《医学衷中参西录》升陷汤（黄芪、柴胡、升麻、桔梗）加人参、山茱萸。

Literature Review of Debilitation of Ancestral Qì

📖 *Chóng Dìng Tōng Sú Shāng Hán Lùn* ("Revised Popular On Cold Damage"), "Vacuity and Repletion of Qì and Blood"

> "Lung qì vacuity results in panting and hasty breathing, intermittent sweating, dry throat and low voice, qì shortage with inability to speak, faint speech, and speaking only at the end of the day."

This quotation describes how lung qì vacuity, debilitation of ancestral qì, and forceless voice cause low voice, qì timidity, and dysphonia.

📖 *Yī Xué Zhōng Zhōng Cān Xī Lù* ("Records of Chinese Medicine with Reference to Western Medicine"), "Formulas for Treating Downward Fall of Great Qì"

> "Great qì is internal qì. The qì of breathing is external qì. When a person feels that the external qì of breathing does not connect with internal qì, this indicates that great qì is vacuous, verging on falling, and unable to tightly embrace the outside of the lung… If this condition is severe, breathing will stop and then begin again only with great strain. People mistakenly think that qì counterflow causes panting, so they downbear it. As a result, the fall is boosted even further and an unfavorable crisis appears immediately."

It also explains:

> "The manifestations of this disease: Shortness of breath, palpitations and fearful throbbing in the heart, profuse dripping sweat, clouded spirit and forgetfulness, trembling voice and stirring body, alternating heat effusion and aversion to cold, fullness and oppression inside the chest, strained breathing like panting, dry throat and thirst, constant yawning, wilted limbs, tendency to hunger after eating, fecal and urinary incontinence, dribbling urinary block and generalized swelling, exhalation with stretched mouth and failure of qì to reach the upper body, anal hernia, incessant descent of blood in women or even counterflow movement of menstrual fluid, and an innumerable variety of pathologic signs."

Great qì is in fact identical with ancestral qì and with lung qì. When great qì falls downward, clear qì fails to ascend. As a result, the essence of grain and water cannot be transported upward to the heart, lung, head, and eyes, and distributed throughout the entire body. The whole body is deprived of nourishment and organ functions are weakened. This can manifest in the numerous miscellaneous signs described above.

文献评述

《重订通俗伤寒论•气血虚实》曰：“肺气虚者，气喘息促，时时汗出，喉燥音低，气少不能言，言而微，终日乃复言。” 论述肺气虚，宗气衰少，无力发音，故声低气怯，发声困难。

《医学衷中参西录•治大气下陷方》曰：“大气者，内气也。呼吸之气，外气也。人觉有呼吸之外气与内气不相接续者，即大气虚而欲陷，不能紧紧包举肺外也。…其剧者，呼吸将停，努力始能呼吸。犹误认为气逆作喘而降之，则陷者益陷，凶危立见矣。”又说:

"其病之现状: 有呼吸短气者，有心中怔忡者，有淋漓大汗者，有神昏健忘者，有声颤身动者，有寒热往来者，有胸中满闷者，有努力呼吸似喘者，有咽干作渴者，有常常呵欠者，有肢体痿废者，有食后易饥者，有二便不禁者，有癃闭身肿者，有张口呼气外出而气不上达，肛门突出者，有女子下血不止者，更有经水逆行者，种种病状实难悉数。"大气即是宗气、肺气，大气下陷，清气不升，使水谷精微不能上输心肺头目、布散全身，全身失养，脏腑功能减弱，则会表现上述诸多复杂的症状。

Summary of Debilitation of Ancestral Qì
1. Dysphonia Low voice and qì timidity, shortage of qì and laziness to speak, breathing with weak qì, cough and panting in a low voice. 2. Qì Failing to Move Blood *Failure to luxuriate the face*: Pale white facial complexion, pale lips and tongue. *Qì vacuity with blood stasis:* Heart palpitations and fearful throbbing, oppression and stifling pain in the chest, dark purple facial complexion, green-blue or purple lips and nails. 3. Downward Fall of Great Qì Shortness of breath, belabored exhalation, faint breathing, fatigue and lack of strength, devitalized essence-spirit, slowness of thought, at critical times sudden stopped breathing.

宗气衰少
发音困难——声低气怯，少气懒言，呼吸气弱，咳喘声低。 气不行血——不荣于面—面色淡白，唇舌色淡。 气虚血瘀—心悸怔忡，胸闷憋痛，面色紫暗，唇甲青紫。 大气下陷——短气，呼出困难，气息微弱，身倦乏力，精神不振，思维迟钝，严重时可见呼吸顿停。

4.6 Lung Qì Verging on Desertion

When insufficiency of lung qì progresses further into severe debilitation, the breathing function is reduced drastically, essential qì in the organs verges on expiry, qì cannot be kept in the inner body, and original qì dissipates and deserts to the outside. This manifests in severe debilitation of the breathing function, which is a critical pathomechanism. Severe vacuity of lung qì disturbs diffusion and downbearing, preventing it from carrying out its function of breathing. In this case, you will observe qì panting and breathing with flaring nostrils, faint and discontinuous breathing, in severe cases sometimes interrupted, and a timid unclear low voice.

When qì fails to nourish the spirit, you will observe haziness of the spirit-affect and in severe cases, stupor. Severe vacuity of lung qì causes external defense to become insecure, so that the interstices lose their tight seal and the fluids are discharged outward. The result is great incessant sweating with pearly sweat. When lung qì is severely vacuous, it fails to propel blood upward to luxuriate the face, which results in a somber white facial complexion. When qì is discharged outward together with humor, yáng qì fails to reach the four limbs. This results in lack of warmth in the four limbs, a faint pulse on the verge of expiry, and in critical life-threatening cases, symptoms of lung qì on the verge of desertion.

This condition is treated by boosting qì, returning yáng, and stemming desertion. The recommended formulas are *dú shēn tāng* (Pure Ginseng Decoction), *shēn fù tāng* (Ginseng and Aconite Decoction), or *shēn fù lóng mǔ tāng* (Ginseng, Aconite, Dragon Bone, and Oyster Shell Decoction) with the addition of *huáng qí* (Astragali Radix).

Dú Shēn Tāng 独参汤 (Pure Ginseng Decoction)
rén shēn 人参 (Ginseng Radix, ginseng)

Shēn Fù Tāng 人参附子汤 (Ginseng and Aconite Decoction)
rén shēn 人参 (Ginseng Radix, ginseng) *fù zǐ* 制附子 (Aconiti Radix Lateralis Praeparata, processed aconite)

Shēn Fù Lóng Mǔ Tāng 参附龙牡汤 (Ginseng, Aconite, Dragon Bone, and Oyster Shell Decoction)
rén shēn 人参 (Ginseng Radix, ginseng) *fù zǐ* 制附子 (Aconiti Radix Lateralis Praeparata, processed aconite) *lóng gǔ* (Mastodi Ossis Fossilia) *mǔ lì* 牡蛎 (Ostreae Concha, oyster shell) Plus: *huáng qí* 黄耆 (Astragali Radix, astragalus)

肺气欲脱

肺气不足，进一步发展，肺气大衰，呼吸功能极度低下，脏腑精气濒临欲绝，气不能内守，元气涣散，向外脱失，出现呼吸功能严重衰败的危重病机。肺气大虚，宣降失司，不能行使呼吸之职，可见气喘息鼻张，呼吸微弱不续、甚或时有中断、语声低怯不清。气不养神，则见神情淡漠，甚则昏迷。肺气大虚，卫外不固，腠理失密，津液外泄，则大汗不止，汗出如珠。肺气大虚，不能推动血脉，上荣于面，则见面色苍白；气随液泄，阳气不达四肢，则四肢不温、脉微欲绝，呈现肺气欲脱，生命垂危的危重病象。治宜益气回阳固脱。方选独参汤、参附汤、或参附龙牡汤（人参、附子、龙骨、牡蛎）加黄芪。

Literature Review of Lung Qì Verging on Desertion

📖 *Qiān Jīn Yào Fāng* ("A Thousand Gold Pieces Prescriptions"), "Treatise on Lung Pulse"

> "Qì expiry in hand greater yīn results in parched skin and body hair. Greater yīn is what moves qì and warms the skin and body hair. When qì fails to luxuriate, the skin and body hair are parched; when the skin and body hair are parched, the fluids leave; and when the fluids leave, the nodes in the skin are damaged. Damage to the nodes of the skin causes desiccated skin and brittle hair, which means that qì has already died."

It further explains:

> "Lung expiry causes death after three days. How can we know this? An extended mouth but with qì failing to be outthrust, and a white face and green-blue eyes, this is what is called disordered channels."

This quotation points out that expiry of lung qì with original qì verging on desertion can cause symptoms such as parched dry skin and brittle hair. At the same time, it describes that lung qì verging on desertion can very quickly lead to death when critical signs appear, such as stretched mouth with shortness of breath.

📖 *Yī Zōng Jīn Jiàn* ("The Golden Mirror of Medicine"), "Heart Approach to Miscellaneous Diseases in Rhyme; Rapid Panting as a Sign of Impending Death"

> "Panting with moistening from sweat means lung expiry. When the pulse is rough and the limbs are cold, life is in danger. Panting and cough, blood ejection, inability to lie down, and a debilitated body and large pulse mean that great qì has in most cases collapsed."

This quotation describes the cause and pulse signs of lung qì debilitation.

文献评述

《千金要方•肺藏脉论:“手太阴气绝则皮毛焦，太阴者行气温皮毛者也。气弗营则皮毛焦，皮毛焦则津液去，津液去则皮节伤，皮节伤者，则皮枯毛折，毛折者，则气先死。”又说:“肺绝三日死，何以知之？口张但气出不还，面白目青，是谓乱经。”指出肺气衰绝，元气欲脱，可致皮毛焦枯，毛折等症。同时论述肺气欲脱，出现张口短气等危重症状，很快就会死亡。

《医宗金鉴•杂病心法要诀•喘急死证:“喘汗润发为肺绝，脉涩肢寒命不昌，喘咳吐血不得卧，形衰脉大气多亡。”阐述了肺气衰微的诱发原因和脉症。

Summary of Lung Qì Verging on Desertion

1. Faint Breathing

   Panting and breathing with flaring nostrils, weakened and possibly interrupted breathing, timid unclear low voice.

2. Qì Failing to Nourish the Spirit

   Haziness of the spirit-affect, with stupor in severe cases.

3. Insecurity of External Defense

   Incessant profuse sweating, putting forth pearly sweat.

4. Qì and Blood Failing to Luxuriate

   Somber white facial complexion, lack of warmth in the limbs, faint pulse verging on expiry.

肺气欲脱

气息微弱——喘息鼻张，呼吸微弱，时或中断、低怯不清。

气不养神——神情淡漠，甚则昏迷。

卫外不固——大汗不止，汗出如珠。

气血失荣——面色苍白、四肢不温、脉微欲绝。

Severe Lung Qi Vacuity Pathomechanisms

When the pathomechanism of lung qì vacuity progresses to a more advanced state, it can cause a variety of pathomechanical changes.

Dual Vacuity of Lung Qì and Lung Yáng

When lung qì is vacuous, its functions of promoting movement, stimulating and effusing, and warming can be reduced and vacuity cold can arise internally. This leads to a vacuity of lung yáng and consequently to the appearance of the pathomechanisms of dual vacuity of lung qì and lung yáng. In clinic, we observe signs like shortage of qì and shortness of breath, physical cold and cold limbs, and thin clear phlegm-drool. This condition is treated by supplementing and boosting qì and yáng. The recommended formula is *bǎo yuán tāng* (Origin-Preserving Decoction) from the *Jǐng Yuè Quán Shū* ("Jǐng-Yuè's Complete Compendium").

Bǎo Yuán Tāng 保元汤 (Origin-Preserving Decoction)
rén shēn 人参 (Ginseng Radix, ginseng) *huáng qí* 黄芪 (Astragali Radix, astragalus) *guì zhī* 桂枝 (Cinnamomi Ramulus, cinnamon twig) *gān cǎo* 甘草 (Glycyrrhizae Radix, licorice)

Dual Vacuity of Lung Qì and Lung Yīn

When lung qì is vacuous, engenderment and transformation is insufficient, qì fails to transform yīn, and yīn humor is depleted. This can develop into lung yīn vacuity and advance further into dual vacuity of lung qì and lung yīn. In clinic, we observe signs like shortage of qì and shortness of breath, dry cough with scant phlegm, and vexing heat in the five hearts. This condition is treated by double supplementation of qì and yáng. The recommended formula is *shēng mài sǎn* (Pulse-Engendering Powder) from the *Nèi Wài Shāng Biàn Huò* ("Problem Solving in Internal and External Damage").

Shēng Mài Sǎn 生脉散 (Pulse-Engendering Powder)
rén shēn 人参 (Ginseng Radix, ginseng) *mài mén dōng* 麦门冬 (Ophiopogonis Radix, ophiopogon) *wǔ wèi zǐ* 五味子 (Schisandrae Fructus, schisandra)

Lung-Heart Qì Vacuity

The chapter, "Various Formulas for Treating Lung Congestion Heat" in the *Tài Píng Shèng Huì Fāng* ("The Great Peace Sagacious Benevolence Formulary") states: "The lung lives above the diaphragm and in close proximity to the heart. The heart governs blood, and the lung governs qì. When qì and blood are in harmony with each other, they circulate through the exterior and interior." This source explains the close relationship between the lung governing qì and the heart governing blood. If lung qì vacuity is prolonged and qì vacuity becomes rather severe, it will invariably also cause vacuity of ancestral qì and prevent it from assisting the heart in moving blood. Heart qì degenerates day by day, which can progress into heart qì vacuity.

When the heart and lung share a disease, this results in the pathomechanism of lung-heart qì vacuity. In clinic, we observe signs like shortage of qì and shortness of breath, heart palpitations, and purple lips and green-blue face. This condition is treated by supplementing and boosting heart and lung qì. The recommended formula is *bǔ fèi tāng* (Lung-Supplementing Decoction) from the *Yǒng Lèi Líng Fāng* ("Previously Published Formulas For The Benefit Of All Posterity"), in combination with *bǎo yuán tāng* (Origin-Preserving Decoction) from the *Jǐng Yuè Quán Shū* ("Jǐng-Yuè's Complete Compendium").

Bǔ Fèi Tāng 补肺汤 (Lung-Supplementing Decoction)
rén shēn 人参 (Ginseng Radix, ginseng)
huáng qí 黄芪 (Astragali Radix, astragalus)
shú dì huáng 熟地黄 (Rehmanniae Radix Praeparata, cooked rehmannia)
wǔ wèi zǐ 五味子 (Schisandrae Fructus, schisandra)
zǐ wǎn 紫菀 (Asteris Radix, aster)
sāng bái pí 桑白皮 (Mori Cortex, mulberry root bark)

Bǎo Yuán Tāng 保元汤 (Origin-Preserving Decoction)
rén shēn 人参 (Ginseng Radix, ginseng)
huáng qí 黄芪 (Astragali Radix, astragalus)
guì zhī 桂枝 (Cinnamomi Ramulus, cinnamon twig)
gān cǎo 甘草 (Glycyrrhizae Radix, licorice)

Lung-Spleen Qì Vacuity

The lung governs the qì of the entire body, and the spleen is the source of blood and qì formation. Thus, both viscera are closely related to qì formation. When lung qì is vacuous, the child can steal the mother's qì, and spleen qì can also become vacuous. Failure of lung qì to assist the spleen in movement and transformation and impaired splenic movement and transformation can lead to the pathomechanism of lung-spleen qì vacuity. In clinic, we observe signs like shortage of qì with insufficiency in breathing, low voice, and laziness to speak, occurring simultaneously with torpid intake and reduced eating, and abdominal distention after eating. This condition is treated by boosting qì and fortifying the spleen.

The recommended formula is *liù jūn zǐ tāng* (Six Gentlemen Decoction) from the *Fù Rén Liáng Fāng* ("Good Remedies for Women").

Liù Jūn Zǐ Tāng 六君子汤 (Six Gentlemen Decoction)
rén shēn 人参 (Ginseng Radix, ginseng)
fú líng 茯苓 (Poria, poria)
bái zhú 白术 (Atractylodis Macrocephalae Rhizoma, white atractylodes)
bàn xià 半夏 (Pinelliae Rhizoma, pinellia)
chén pí 陈皮 (Citri Reticulatae Pericarpium, tangerine peel)
gān cǎo 甘草 (Glycyrrhizae Radix, licorice)

Lung-Kidney Qì Vacuity

The lung is the governor of qì, and the kidney is the root of qì. If lung qì is vacuous for a long period of time, it becomes unable to move essence to enrich the kidney, thereby affecting the root. Kidney qì can also become vacuous. When the lung fails to govern the exhalation of qì and the kidney fails to govern the absorption of qì, this can develop into the pathomechanism of lung-kidney qì vacuity. In clinic, we observe signs like enduring cough and panting, shallow breathing, shortness of breath and difficulty in breathing continuously, and severe panting during physical activity. This condition is treated by supplementing and boosting lung and kidney qì. The recommended formula is *rén shēn gé jiè sǎn* (Ginseng and Gecko Powder) from the *Wèi Shēng Bǎo Jiàn* ("Precious Mirror of Health") in combination with *qī wèi dū qì wán* (Seven-Ingredient Metropolis Qì Pill) from the *Yī Zōng Jǐ Rèn Biān* ("Transmission of Medical Orthodoxy"), which is *liù wèi dì huáng tāng* (Six-Ingredient Rehmannia Decoction) with the addition of *wǔ wèi zǐ* (Schisandrae Fructus).

Rén Shēn Gé Jiè Sǎn 人参蛤蚧散 (Ginseng and Gecko Powder)
gé jiè 蛤蚧 (Gecko, gecko)
xìng rén 杏仁 (Armeniacae Semen, apricot kernel)
gān cǎo 甘草 (Glycyrrhizae Radix, licorice)
rén shēn 人参 (Ginseng Radix, ginseng)
fú líng 茯苓 (Poria, poria)
bèi mǔ 贝母 (Fritillariae Bulbus, fritillaria)
sāng bái pí 桑白皮 (Mori Cortex, mulberry root bark)
zhī mǔ 知母 (Anemarrhenae Rhizoma, anemarrhena)

Qī Wèi Dū Qì Wán 七味都气丸 (Seven-Ingredient Metropolis Qì Pill)
shú dì huáng 熟地黄 (Rehmanniae Radix Praeparata, cooked rehmannia) *shān zhū yú* 山茱萸 (Corni Fructus, cornus) *shān yào* 山药 (Dioscoreae Rhizoma, dioscorea) *zé xiè* 泽泻 (Alismatis Rhizoma, alisma) *mǔ dān pí* 牡丹皮 (Moutan Cortex, moutan) *fú líng* 茯苓 (Poria, poria) *wǔ wèi zǐ* 五味子 (Schisandrae Fructus, schisandra)

肺气虚的病机进一步发展，可引起多种病机变化。

肺的气阳两虚: 肺气虚，推动、激发、温煦的功能减弱，虚寒内生，可引起肺的阳虚，从而出现肺气肺阳同时兼虚的病机。临床可见少气短息，形寒肢冷，痰涎清稀等症。治宜补益气阳，方选《景岳全书》保元汤。

肺的气阴两虚: 肺气虚，生化不足，气不化阴，阴液亏损，可发展为肺阴虚，进而形成肺的气阴两虚。临床可见少气短息，干咳痰少，五心烦热等症。治宜气阳双补。方选《内外伤辨惑》生脉散。

肺心气虚: 《太平圣惠方•治肺脏壅热诸方》云: “夫肺居膈上，与心脏相近，心主于血，肺主于气，气血相和，循环表里。”说明肺主气与心主血有密切的关系。若肺气虚日久，气虚较甚，势必宗气亦虚，不能助心行血，心气日溃，进而引起心气亦虚，肺心同病，引起肺心气虚的病机。临床可见气短喘息，心悸，唇紫面青等症。治宜补益心肺之气。方选《永类钤方》补肺汤合《景岳全书》保元汤。

肺脾气虚: 肺主一身之气，脾为气血生化之源，二脏与气的生成有密切关系，肺气虚，子盗母气，脾气亦虚，肺气不能助脾运化，脾失健运，可引起肺脾气虚的病机。临床先见少气不足以息，声低懒言，同时伴见纳呆食少，食后腹胀等症。治宜益气健脾。方选《妇人良方》六君子汤。

肺肾气虚: 肺为气之主，肾为气之根，若肺气虚日久，不能输精以滋肾，累及根本，肾气亦虚，肺不主呼气，肾不主纳气，可发展为肺肾气虚的病机。临床可见久病咳喘。呼吸表浅，气短难续，动则喘甚等症。治宜补益肺肾之气。方选《卫生宝鉴》人参蛤蚧散合《医宗己任编》七味都气丸（六味地黄汤加五味子）。

Chapter Five

Lung Yáng Vacuity

The *Huáng Dì Nèi Jīng* ("The Yellow Emperor's Inner Canon") does not directly mention lung yáng vacuity by name, but its discussion of lung vacuity and lung cold already includes the pathomechanism of lung yáng vacuity. For example, the chapter, "Channel Vessels" in the *Líng Shū* ("The Magic Pivot") states: "The lung is associated with the hand greater yīn vessel...Vacuity of its qì results in pain and cold in the shoulder and back, shortage of qì and insufficiency in breathing, and changes in the color of urine." This is the earliest record of the pattern of lung yáng vacuity.

The chapter, "Pulse Symptoms and Treatments of Lung Wilting, Lung Welling-Abscess, Cough, and Qì Ascent" in the *Jīn Guì Yào Lüe* ("Essential Prescriptions of the Golden Coffer") explains:

> "In lung wilting with drool foaming at the mouth but without cough, the patient will not be thirsty but invariably suffer from enuresis and frequent urination. The reason for this is that vacuity in the upper body prevents it from controlling the lower body. This indicates cold inside the lung and is invariably accompanied by dizziness and increased drool and spittle. Use *gān cǎo gān jiāng tāng* (Licorice and Dried Ginger Decoction) to warm it."

In this quotation, Zháng Zhòng-Jǐng still does not mention lung yáng vacuity by name, but nevertheless includes a description of cold inside the lung, which is very similar to the pathomechanism of lung yáng vacuity.

The chapter, "Lung Vacuity Cold" in the *Qiān Jīn Yào Fāng* ("A Thousand Gold Pieces Prescriptions") stated: "When a person suffers from shortage of qi, insufficiency in breathing, and dry throat without fluids, this is called lung vacuity cold." In the *Wài Tái Mì Yào* ("Essential Secrets from Outside the Metropolis"), Wáng Tāo clearly pointed out that the signs of lung vacuity cold are "a hoarse and congested voice, panting and exhausted breathing, and cough with spittle." Zhāng Sān-Xī indicated in the *Zhì Fǎ Huì* ("Collected Methods of Treatment") that the symptom of cough, when caused by "vacuity cold inside the lung," was characterized by "coughing of white phlegm, white foam, ... sweet taste in the mouth, and drool foaming and running." The chapter, "Internal Damage Swelling" in the *Zhèng Yīn Mài Zhì* ("Pathoconditions: Causes, Pulses, and Treatments") stated: "Lung vacuity water swelling ... manifests in a deathly pale facial complexion, uninhibited clear stool and urine, and qì timidity and departure of the spirit. This indicates a vacuity of the lung's true yáng." All these sources analyze in depth the pathomechanical changes caused by lung yáng vacuity.

More recently, Táng Róng-Chuān directly mentioned the term "liver yáng vacuity" in a commentary on the *Jīn Guì Yào Lüè* ("Essential Prescriptions of the Golden Coffer"). His *Jīn Guì Yào Lüè Qiǎn* ("Simple Commentaries and Corrections to the 'Essential Prescriptions of the Golden Coffer'") explains in the chapter, "Pulse Symptoms and Treatments of Lung Wilting, Pulmonary Welling-Abscess, Cough, and Qì Ascent":

> "A patient with drool foaming at the mouth but no coughing or thirst is bound to suffer from enuresis and frequent urination, since lung yáng is vacuous and unable to control the lower body. This indicates cold inside the lung and *gān cǎo gān jiāng tāng* (Licorice and Dried Ginger Decoction) is suitable for warming it."

In the chapter, "Seeking the Root in Pattern Identification" in the *Pú Fǔ Zhōu Yī Liáo Jīng Yàn* ("Pú Fǔ-Zhōu's Medical Experience"), the famous clinician Pú Fǔ-Zhōu emphasized even more prominently the clinical application of lung yáng vacuity, which has caused it to achieve wide-spread attention. In the past seventy or eighty years an extensive and in-depth dispute has taken place in the national journals, as a result of which the pathomechanism of lung yáng vacuity has gradually become recognized by the overall profession.

Among the causes of lung yáng vacuity, the most important is prolonged lodging of external evil in the lung viscus, in particular in the form of an invasion of cold-damp evil into the lung that damages yáng qì, as is referred to in the expression "a cold body and drinking fluids damages the lung." In addition, lung yáng vacuity can gradually evolve from lung qì vacuity that is caused by prolonged cough or panting consuming lung qì. Lastly, excessive taxation wearing on qì over a long period can damage yáng, or a yáng vacuity in other bowels and viscera can spread to the lung. The pathomechanical changes of lung yáng vacuity can be differentiated into four aspects: lung cold with loss of warmth; lung cold with collecting liquid; lung cold with congealing blood; and lung cold with loss of restraint.

肺阳虚

《黄帝内经》虽未正式提出肺阳虚的名称，但从论及肺虚、肺寒的概念中已包含着肺阳虚的病机。如《灵枢•经脉》云："肺手太阴之脉，…气虚则肩背痛寒，少气不足以息，溺色变。"是肺阳虚证的最早记载。《金匮要略•肺痿肺痈咳嗽上气病脉证治》说："肺痿吐涎沫而不咳者，其人不渴，必遗尿，小便数。所以然者，以上虚不能制下故也。此为肺中冷，必眩，多涎唾，甘草干姜汤以温之。"仲景仍未提出肺阳虚的名称，却有肺中冷的论述，与肺阳虚的病机大体相似。《千金要方•肺虚冷》"病苦少气，不足以息，嗌干不津液，名曰肺虚冷。" 王焘《外台秘要》明确指出肺虚寒可见"声音嘶塞，气息喘惫，咳唾"症状。张三锡《治法汇》指出："肺中虚寒"所致咳嗽的症状特点为"咳白痰，作白泡，…口甘，涎沫流。"《症因脉治•内伤肿胀》"肺虚水肿，…如面色惨白，二便清利，气怯神离，肺之真阳虚也。"均对肺阳虚所致病机变化作了深入探讨。直到近代唐容川在《金匮要略》注释时，才正式提出"肺阳虚"的名称。如《金匮要略浅注补正•肺痿肺痈咳嗽上气》说："吐涎沫而不咳者，又不渴，必遗尿，小便数，以肺阳虚不能制下，此为肺中冷，…宜甘草干姜汤以温之。"著名临床家蒲辅周在《蒲辅周医疗经验•辨证求本》中更为突出地强调了肺阳虚的临床应用，从而引起大家的普遍重视。七、八十年代以来，国内期刊杂志上展开了广泛而深入的争论，肺阳虚的病机才逐渐被大家公认。引起肺阳虚的病因主要有外邪久恋肺脏，特别是寒湿之邪犯肺，损伤阳气，所谓"形寒饮冷则伤肺"是也；亦可因久咳久喘，耗伤肺气，由肺气虚渐致肺阳虚；亦有过劳耗气，日久伤阳，或由它脏阳虚，波及于肺。肺阳虚的病机变化可分为肺寒失温，肺寒津停，肺寒血凝和肺寒失制等四个方面。

5.1 Lung Cold with Loss of Warmth

Lung yáng has the function of warming the lung connector. When lung yáng is debilitated, it loses its ability to warm. Congealing cold and contracting qì cause the lobes of the lung to contract, blocking instead of stretching them. They also obstruct the qì dynamic and impair diffusion and downbearing. This manifests as cough, panting, and oppression in the chest and is treated by warming the lung, boosting qì, and dissipating cold. The recommended formula is *bǔ fèi tāng* (Lung-Supplementing Decoction) from the *Sān Yīn Jí Yī Bìng Zhèng Fāng Lùn* ("A Unified Treatise on Diseases, Patterns, and Remedies According to the Three Causes").

Bǔ Fèi Tāng 补肺汤 (Lung-Supplementing Decoction)
rén shēn 人参 (Ginseng Radix, ginseng)
ròu guì 肉桂 (Cinnamomi Cortex, cinnamon bark)
yáng qǐ shí 阳起石 (Actinolitum, actinolite)
zhōng rǔ fěn 钟乳粉 (Stalactitum Pulveratum, powdered stalactite)
sāng bái pí 桑白皮 (Mori Cortex, mulberry root bark)
zǐ wǎn 紫菀 (Asteris Radix, aster)
kuǎn dōng huā 款冬花 (Farfarae Flos, coltsfoot)
wǔ wèi zǐ 五味子 (Schisandrae Fructus, schisandra)
mài mén dōng 麦门冬 (Ophiopogonis Radix, ophiopogon)

When lung yáng is depleted, its stimulating and propelling function is weakened. The result is shallow breathing, no strength to inhale the clear and expel the turbid, weakened and accelerated breathing with a low sound, and then shortness of breath, shortage of qì, and a low timid voice. The chapter, "Vacuity Taxation and Shortage of Qì" in the *Zhū Bìng Yuán Hòu Lùn* ("The Origin and Indicators of Disease") explains: "Damage to the lung from vacuity taxation results in shortage of qì. The lung governs qì, and qì is yáng. This is the reason for insufficiency of yáng qì." This quotation directly illustrates how a vacuity of yáng qì in the lung can lead to shortage of qì. This condition is treated by warming the lung and boosting qì. The recommended formula is *wēn fèi tāng* (Lung-Warming Decoction).

Wēn Fèi Tāng 温肺汤 (Lung-Warming Decoction)
rén shēn 人参 (Ginseng Radix, ginseng)
zhōng rǔ fěn 钟乳粉 (Stalactitum Pulveratum, powdered stalactite)
ròu guì 肉桂 (Cinnamomi Cortex, cinnamon bark)
gān jiāng 干姜 (Zingiberis Rhizoma, dried ginger)
shēng jiāng 生姜 (Zingiberis Rhizoma Recens, fresh ginger)
bàn xià 半夏 (Pinelliae Rhizoma, pinellia)
jú hóng 橘红 (Citri Reticulatae Exocarpium Rubrum, red tangerine peel)
mù xiāng 木香 (Aucklandiae Radix, costusroot)
zhì gān cǎo 炙甘草 (Glycyrrhizae Radix Praeparata, mix-fried licorice)

When yáng is unable to control yīn as a result of lung yáng vacuity, exuberant internal yīn cold impairs the diffusion of defense yáng to warm the fleshy exterior and fatten the interstices. As a result, the skin is deprived of warmth and nourishment, which manifests in fear of cold and liking for warmth, fear of cold in the shoulder and back, cold extremities, and parched skin and body hair. When defense yáng is debilitated, the fleshy exterior is insecure and therefore unable to fight against external evil. The result is spontaneous sweating and recurring contractions of the common cold. This condition is treated by warming the lung and dissipating cold, and by boosting qì and securing the exterior. The recommended formula is *gān cǎo gān jiāng tāng* (Licorice and Dried Ginger Decoction) from the *Jīn Guì Yào Lüè* ("Essential Prescriptions of the Golden Coffer"), in combination with *yù píng fēng sǎn* (Jade Wind-Barrier Powder) from the *Dān Xī Xīn Fǎ* ("Dān Xī's Heart-Approach").

Gān Cǎo Gān Jiāng Tāng 甘草干姜汤 (Licorice and Dried Ginger Decoction)
gān cǎo 甘草 (Glycyrrhizae Radix, licorice) *gān jiāng* 干姜 (Zingiberis Rhizoma, dried ginger)

Yù Píng Fēng Sǎn 玉屏风散 (Jade Wind-Barrier Powder)
huáng qí 黄芪 (Astragali Radix, astragalus) *bái zhú* 白术 (Atractylodis Macrocephalae Rhizoma, white atractylodes) *fáng fēng* 防风 (Saposhnikoviae Radix, saposhnikovia)

The chapter, "Lung Taxation" in the *Qiān Jīn Yào Fāng* ("A Thousand Gold Pieces Prescriptions") explains: "Lung taxation vacuity cold … causes qì ascent, fullness in the chest, panting, and qì expiry." The chapter, "Discussing Treatment of Vacuity and Repletion in the Lung and Large Intestine" in the *Yán Shì Jì Shēng Fāng* ("Yan's Remedies for Curing All People") also explains:

> "If the lung is vacuous, vacuity engenders cold, and cold results in hoarse voice, strained speech, trembling and weakness, insufficiency of qì, completely dry throat, vacuity cold with lack of qì, fear and unhappiness, cough to the point of panting, clear snivel in the nose, parched skin and body hair, and a pulse that manifests as sunken and moderate. All these are symptoms of lung vacuity."

When these sources refer to vacuity cold, it means that lung yáng is vacuous and fails to warm. The chapter, "Seeking the Root in Pattern Identification" in the *Pú Fǔ Zhōu Yī Liáo Jīng Yàn* ("Pú Fǔ-Zhōu's Medical Experience") states even more clearly: "Lung yáng vacuity results in susceptibility to the common cold, because defense qì is vacuous and resistance is weakened."

肺寒失温

肺阳有温煦肺系的作用。肺阳虚衰，失却温煦，寒凝气缩，肺叶收敛，闭而不张，气机受阻，宣降失职，发为咳嗽、气喘、胸闷。治宜温肺益气散寒。方选《三因极一病证方论》补肺汤（人参、桂心、白石英、钟乳粉、桑白皮、紫菀、冬花、五味子、麦冬）；肺阳亏虚，振奋、推动功能减弱，呼吸表浅，无力吸清排浊，呼吸气息微弱，频率加快，声息降低，则为气短少气，声音低怯。《诸病源候论•虚劳少气》说：“虚劳伤于肺，故少气。肺主气，气为阳，此为阳气不足故也。”直接阐明肺的阳气虚衰可致少气。治宜温肺益气。方选温肺汤（人参、钟乳石、肉桂、干姜、生姜、半夏、橘红、木香、炙甘草）；肺阳虚衰，阳不制阴，阴寒内盛，不能宣发卫阳以温煦肌表，肥厚腠理，肌肤失温、失养，则为畏寒喜暖、肩背怕冷、手足寒冷、皮毛焦枯。卫阳虚衰，肌表不固，不能抗御外邪，则为自汗、反复感冒。治宜温肺散寒，益气固表。方选《金匮要略》甘草干姜汤合《丹溪心法》玉屏风散。《千金要方•肺劳》说：“肺劳虚冷，…上气，胸满，喘息气绝。”《济生方•肺大肠虚实论治》也说：“方其虚也，虚则生寒，寒则声嘶，语言用力，颤掉缓弱，少气不足，咽中干无津液，虚寒乏气，恐布不乐，咳嗽及喘，鼻有清涕，皮毛焦枯，诊其脉沉缓者，是肺虚之候也。”文中虚冷、虚寒，均指肺阳虚失于温煦。《蒲辅周医疗经验•辨证求本》更明确指出：“肺阳虚，则易感冒，因卫气虚，抵抗力弱。”

Literature Review of Lung Cold with Loss of Warmth

🕮 *Qiān Jīn Yào Fāng* (“A Thousand Gold Pieces Prescriptions”), “Treatise on Lung Pulse; on Lung Vacuity Cold”

> “When the pulse in the front at the inch, or qì, opening on the right wrist indicates yīn vacuity, this is the hand greater yīn channel. The patient will suffer from shortage of qì and insufficiency in breathing, and completely dry throat. This is called lung vacuity cold.”

It also explains:

> “Insufficiency of lung qì manifests in qì counterflow, fullness, and ascent, oppression and congestion in the throat, and shortness of breath.”

Lung vacuity cold thus means that lung yáng is debilitated and yīn cold exuberant. Since yáng loses its ability to warm and to propel forcefully, breathing is faint and lung qì ascends counterflow, resulting in shortage of qì, shortness of breath, and dyspnea.

🕮 *Lèi Jīng Fù Yì* (“Wings to the Classified Canon”), “Record on Seeking Rightness”

> “Cold cough with vacuity panting and a cool body with spontaneous sweating are caused by yáng vacuity in the viscus of metal, which prevents it from safeguarding the lung.”

Yáng vacuity in the viscus of metal refers precisely to lung yáng vacuity. As a result, the skin loses warmth and is unable to secure external defense, which causes generalized fear of cold and spontaneous incessant sweating.

📖 *Zá Bìng Guǎng Yào* ("Broad Essentials of Miscellaneous Disease"), "Cough"

> "Every single pattern of taxation cough is caused by lung vacuity… The lung governs qì and is reflected in the skin and body hair. Qì vacuity causes slight cold to lodge in the skin and body hair. When this damages a person's lung, the result is insufficiency, which manifests in cough. When qì receives warmth, it perfuses and harmonizes; when it receives cold, it is blocked and rough. Vacuity results in qì being insufficient and therefore distressed by cold. They combine and collect inside the lung, from where they cannot be effused. This causes cough and shortness of breath."

This quotation describes how lung qì vacuity and contraction of cold cause lung qì stagnation and impaired diffusion and downbearing, which can lead to cough and shortness of breath.

📖 *Lín Zhèng Zhǐ Nán Yī Àn* ("A Clinical Guide with Case Histories"), "Cough"

> "Prolonged cough that persists over a number of years, cold back and constant cold in the instep, copious white sweat, and cough that is so severe that the person is unable to lie down indicate that yáng is debilitated and defense is thin, so that external evil can hit easily and turbid yīn with rheum can invade the upper body. I suggest treatment by harmonizing construction and defense, concurrent with safeguarding yáng. Use *huáng qí jiàn zhōng tāng* (Astragalus Center-Fortifying Decoction) minus *yí táng* (Maltosum), but with *fù zǐ* (Aconiti Radix Lateralis Praeparata) and *fú líng* (Poria) added."

Recurring cough damages lung yáng. Loss of warmth results in physical cold and cold limbs. Insecurity of defense yáng and failure to seal the interstices results in spontaneous sweating. Failure of yáng qì to warm qì and blood and to ascend to luxuriate the face results in a white face. Therefore, one can achieve excellent results by harmonizing construction and defense and warming and supplementing lung yáng.

文献评述

《千金要方•肺脏脉论•肺虚冷》曰: "右手寸口气口以前脉阴虚者，手太阴经也。病苦少气不足以息，嗌干不津液，名曰肺虚冷也。"又说"肺气不足，逆满上气，咽中闷塞，短气。"肺虚冷，则是肺阳虚衰，阴寒内盛。阳失温煦，推动无力，故气息微弱，肺气上逆而少气、短气，呼吸困难。

《类经附翼•求正录》曰:“寒嗽虚喘，身凉自汗，以金脏之阳虚，不能保肺也。”金脏阳虚，就是肺阳虚，肌表失温，不能卫外为固，则全身畏寒怕冷，自汗不止。

《杂病广要•咳嗽》曰:“劳嗽一证，皆因肺虚，…肺主气，候皮毛，气虚为微寒客皮毛，人伤于肺则不足，成咳嗽。夫气得温则宣和，得寒则否涩。虚则气不足而为寒所迫，并聚于肺间，不得宣发，故令咳而短气也。”论述肺气虚，受寒而肺气凝滞，失于宣降，可致咳嗽、气短。

《临证指南医案•咳嗽》曰:“久嗽经年，背寒足跗常冷，汗多色白，嗽甚不得卧，此阳微卫薄，外邪易触，而浊阴挟饮上犯，议和营卫，兼护其阳，黄芪建中汤去饴糖加附子茯苓。”反复咳嗽，肺阳损伤，失于温煦，则形寒肢冷；卫阳失固，肌腠失密，则自汗；阳气不能温煦气血，上荣于面，则面白。故用调和营卫，温补肺阳之法而获良效。

Summary of Lung Cold with Loss of Warmth
1. Cold Congealing Lung Qì and Impairing Diffusion and Downbearing Cough, panting, oppression in the chest. 2. Reduced Propelling and Shallow Breathing Shortness of breath with shortage of qì, low weak voice. 3. Impaired Diffusion of Defense Yáng and Impaired Warming of the Fleshy Exterior Fear of cold and liking for warmth, fear of cold in the shoulder and back, cold extremities, parched skin and body hair. 4. Debilitation of Defense Yáng and Insecurity of the Fleshy Exterior Spontaneous sweating, recurring contractions of the common cold.

肺寒失温
寒凝肺气、宣降失职——咳嗽，气喘，胸闷。 推动减弱、呼吸表浅——气短少气，声音低弱。 卫阳失宣、肌表失温——畏寒喜暖，肩背怕冷，手足寒冷，皮毛焦枯。 卫阳虚衰、肌表不固——自汗，反复感冒。

5.2 Lung Cold with Collecting Liquid

The lung governs regulation of the waterways, and lung yáng is able to stimulate its functions of diffusion and depurative downbearing. When yáng distributes harmoniously, qì is transformed, liquid moves, and the fluids are distributed throughout the body, moving equally in all five channels. When lung qì is vacuous and cold, however, debilitated yáng qì is unable to ascend and outthrust through the nose, and the qì of turbid yīn fails to bear downward, asphyxiating and blocking the nose instead. Alternatively, lung yáng vacuity can prevent it from distributing liquid, so that the fluids collect in the nose. Both these can lead to deep-source nasal congestion, manifesting as clear, profuse, incessant snivel, itchy nose, a reduced sense of smell, and not smelling anything but fishy odors.

This condition is treated by warming and supplementing lung qì. The recommended formula is a variation of *wēn fèi zhǐ liú dān* (Lung-Warming Nose-Drying Elixir) from the *Biàn Zhèng Lù* ("Records on Pattern Differentiation").

Wēn Fèi Zhǐ Liú Dān 温肺止流丹 (Lung-Warming Nose-Drying Elixir)
rén shēn 人参 (Ginseng Radix, ginseng)
xì xīn 细辛 (Asari Radix, asarum)
hē zǐ 诃子 (Chebulae Fructus, chebule)
jié gěng 桔梗 (Platycodonis Radix, platycodon)
yú nǎo gāo 鱼脑膏 (Fish Brain Paste)

Zài Yuán-Lǐ mentioned in the *Zhèng Zhì Yào Jué* ("Essential Rhymes for Patterns and Treatment") that clear snivel in the nose that is caused by cold in the brain and lung should be treated with warming medicinals like *xì xīn* (细辛 Asari Radix, asarum), *wū tóu* (Aconiti Radix Wutou), *fù zǐ* (Aconiti Radix Lateralis Praeparata), and *gān jiāng* (Zingiberis Rhizoma). When lung yáng is vacuous, yīn cold exuberates internally. Cold governs congealing and stagnation, and the fluids move when they receive warmth and congeal when they encounter cold. Thus, an exuberance of yīn cold can easily lead to fluids collecting in the lung and transforming into water-damp and phlegm-rheum. As a result of debilitated lung yáng, yáng fails to steam upward, qì fails to transform liquid, and liquid fails to bear upward. This manifests in symptoms such as dry mouth and throat, thirst with a liking for hot drinks, and parched skin.

The chapter, "Lung Vacuity Cold" in the *Qiān Jīn Yào Fāng* ("A Thousand Gold Pieces Prescriptions") explains: "A patient [with lung vacuity cold] manifests with shortage of qì, insufficiency in breathing, and completely dry throat." When lung yáng is vacuous, the fluids are not transformed, but collect and become cold rheum. As a result, we see panting and cough, ejection of clear thin phlegm that is copious and white, the appearance of white foam, drool foaming at the mouth, and in severe cases possibly cough and counterflow with propped breathing and inability to lie down. This condition is treated by warming the lung and dissipating cold, and by transforming phlegm and calming panting.

The recommended formula is *líng gān wǔ wèi jiāng xīn bàn xià xìng rén tāng* (Poria, Licorice, Schisandra, Ginger, Asarum, Pinellia, Almond Seed Decoction) from the *Jīn Guì Yào Lüe* ("Essential Prescriptions of the Golden Coffer"), with the addition of *guì zhī* (Cinnamomi Ramulus).

Líng Gān Wǔ Wèi Jiāng Xīn Bàn Xià Xìng Rén Tāng 苓甘五味姜辛半夏杏仁汤 (Poria, Licorice, Schisandra, Ginger, Asarum, Pinellia, and Almond Decoction)
fú líng 茯苓 (Poria, poria)
gān cǎo 甘草 (Glycyrrhizae Radix, licorice)
wǔ wèi zǐ 五味子 (Schisandrae Fructus, schisandra)
gān jiāng 干姜 (Zingiberis Rhizoma, dried ginger)
xì xīn 细辛 (Asari Radix, asarum)
bàn xià 半夏 (Pinelliae Rhizoma, pinellia)
xìng rén 杏仁 (Armeniacae Semen, almond)

If vacuity impedes the outward diffusion and outthrust of lung yáng, yáng qì inside the chest fails to warm the back. This results in symptoms like aversion to cold in a palm-sized area of the back. The "Treatise on Phlegm-Rheum and Lodged Rheum" in the *Yī Mén Fǎ Lǜ* ("Axioms of Medicine") explains this:

> "When people say that 'lodged rheum inside the chest obstructs heart-lung yáng in the upper burner and causes yīn to choke and therefore deeply penetrate into the back,' it means that there is cold but no heat, and this cold is at the same time obstructing the ascent of yáng in the governing vessel. Thus, coldness in a palm-sized area of the back is under all circumstances a sign of internal depression of yáng fire."

This condition is treated by warming the lung and freeing yáng. The recommended formula is *fù zǐ tāng* (Aconite Decoction) from the *Shāng Hán Lùn* ("On Cold Damage").

Fù Zǐ Tāng 附子汤 (Aconite Decoction)
fù zǐ 附子 (Aconiti Radix Lateralis Praeparata, processed aconite)
rén shēn 人参 (Ginseng Radix, ginseng)
fú líng 茯苓 (Poria, poria)
bái zhú 白术 (Atractylodis Macrocephalae Rhizoma, white atractylodes)
sháo yào 芍药 (Paeoniae Radix, peony)

In addition, in his *Yī Mén Fǎ Lǜ* ("Axioms of Medicine"), "Water Swelling," Yù Jiā-Yán explained: "When hand greater yīn lung is sufficient at regulating the waterways into the lower body, the ocean cannot develop large waves." In this citation, Dr. Yù illustrates an important pathomechanism, referring to the fact that the lung's yáng qì has the function of steaming, transforming, and spreading the fluids, thereby preventing the flooding of water qì and the formation of water swelling. When lung yáng in the upper burner is depleted, the fluids that are moved upward by the spleen fail to be steamed and transformed. The lung fails to carry out depuration, and the fluids cannot be transported down into the urinary bladder, but spill into the skin and form water swelling.

The chapter, "Swelling" in the "Schema of Miscellaneous Patterns" in the *Jǐng Yuè Quán Shū* ("Jǐng-Yuè's Complete Compendium") states:

> "Any conditions like water swelling are in fact related to disease of the spleen, lung, and kidney. Water is consummate yīn; its root is therefore in the kidney. Water is transformed by qì; its tip is therefore in the lung... When the lung is vacuous, qì fails to transform essence and water... When there is no yáng within yīn, qì is unable to transform, and therefore the fluids in the waterways are stopped, spill over, and form swelling."

The chapter, "Internal Damage Swelling" in the *Zhèng Yīn Mài Zhì* ("Pathoconditions: Causes, Pulses, and Treatments") also explains:

> "Here is the cause of generalized lung vacuity swelling: Excessive taxation leads to chronic vacuity of lung qì. As a result, depuration is not carried out, and the power to downbear is impaired. Defense qì is congested and trapped, and construction qì is unable to follow. This results in the signs of swelling."

In this quotation, lung qì vacuity in fact already includes the pathomechanism of lung yáng debilitation and disabled qì transformation. Later on, this text states even more succinctly: "Lung vacuity water swelling ...manifests in a deathly pale facial complexion, uninhibited clear stool and urine, and qì timidity and departure of the spirit. This indicates a vacuity of the lung's true yáng." This condition is treated by warming yáng, diffusing the lung, and moving water. The recommended formula is *fáng jǐ huáng qí tāng* (Fangji and Astragalus Decoction) from the *Jīn Guì Yào Lüè* ("Essential Prescriptions of the Golden Coffer") with additions.

Fáng Jǐ Huáng Qí Tāng 防己黄耆汤 (Fangji and Astragalus Decoction)
fáng jǐ 防己 (Stephaniae Tetrandrae Radix, fangji) *huáng qí* 黄耆 (Astragali Radix, astragalus *bái zhú* 白朮 (Atractylodis Macrocephalae Rhizoma, white atractylodes) *gān cǎo* 甘草 (Glycyrrhizae Radix, licorice)

Plus:
guì zhī 桂枝 (Cinnamomi Ramulus, cinnamon twig)
gān jiāng 干姜 (Zingiberis Rhizoma, dried ginger)

肺寒津停

肺主通调水道，肺阳能振奋、激发宣发肃降功能，阳和布敷，气化津行，水津四布，五经并行。肺气虚寒，虚衰之阳气，不能上透鼻窍，致浊阴之气不降，窒塞鼻窍，或肺阳虚不能布津，津液停留鼻窍，均可引起鼻渊，表现为清涕长流不止，不臭而腥，鼻痒，嗅觉减退。治宜温补肺气，方选《辨证录》温肺止流丹（人参、细辛、柯子、桔梗、鱼脑骨）化裁。载原礼《证治要诀》提出脑冷肺寒所致，鼻流清涕，用细辛、乌头、附子、干姜之类温热药进行治疗。肺阳虚，阴寒内盛，寒主凝滞，津液得热则行，遇寒则凝，易致津液停肺，化生水湿痰饮。肺阳虚衰，阳失蒸腾，气不化津，津不上承，则见口燥咽干、渴喜热饮、皮肤焦枯等症。如《千金要方•肺虚冷》说："病苦少气，不足以息，嗌干不津液。"肺阳虚，津液不化，停为寒饮，则见咳嗽气喘、吐痰清稀、量多色白、呈泡沫状、口吐涎沫、甚或咳逆倚息不得卧等症。治宜温肺散寒，化痰平喘。方选《金匮要略》苓甘五味姜辛半夏杏仁汤加桂枝。若阻碍肺阳向外宣达，胸中阳气不暖后背，则见背恶寒如掌大之症。正如《医门法律•痰饮留饮论》说："言胸中留饮，阻遏上焦心肺之阳，而为阴噎，则其深入背者，有冷无热，并阻督脉上升之阳，而背寒如掌大，无非阳火内郁之象也。"治宜温肺通阳。方选《伤寒论》附子汤（附子、人参、茯苓、白术、芍药）；另外，喻嘉言说："手太阴肺，足以通调水道于下，海不扬波矣"（《医门法律•水肿》）。这里喻氏阐述了一个重要病机，即肺之阳气有蒸化布散津液，防止水气泛溢而成水肿的作用。如果上焦肺阳亏虚，由脾上输的津液无以蒸化，肺不行清肃之令，津液不能下输膀胱，泛溢肌肤则成水肿。《景岳全书•杂证膜•肿胀》云："凡水肿等症，乃脾、肺、肾三脏相干之病。盖水为至阴，故其本在肾；水化于气，故其标在肺。…今肺虚，则气不化精而化水。…阴中无阳，则气不能化，所以水道不通，溢而为肿。"《症因脉治•内伤肿胀》亦说："肺虚身肿之因，劳疫过度，肺气久虚，清肃之令不行，下降之权失职，卫气壅遏，营气不从，则肿症作矣。"这里肺气虚，实际已包含肺阳亏虚，气化无能的病机在内。随即更明确指出："肺虚水肿，…如面色惨白，二便清利，气怯神离，肺之真阳虚也。"治宜温阳宣肺行水。方选《金匮要略》防己黄芪汤（防己、黄芪、白术、甘草）加桂枝、干姜。

Literature Review of Lung Cold with Collecting Liquid

📖 *Qiān Jīn Yào Fāng* ("A Thousand Gold Pieces Prescriptions"), "Lung Vacuity and Repletion; Lung Vacuity Cold"

> "Lung cold damage causes qì cough with snivel, spittle, and nasal congestion."

When cold evil damages the lung, it damages lung yáng, stops lung qì, and congests the nose. The fluids congeal and stagnate, resulting in running snivel and spittle.

📖 *Shèng Jì Zǒng Lù* ("Sages' Salvation Records"), "Section on the Lung Viscus"

> "It is said that a weakened lung viscus means damage by wind evil, which results in clear cold qì surging upward causing runny nose with clear snivel. The lung opens at the nose and among the humors, is associated with snivel."

When lung yáng is vacuous, it is unable to distribute liquid, and this transforms into snivel instead. The result is uninterrupted clear snivel.

📖 *Biàn Zhèng Lù* ("Records of Pattern Differentiation"), "Deep-Source Nasal Congestion"

> "When a person suffers from runny nose with clear snivel that is prolonged for years without recovery, it means lung qì vacuity cold."

It further explains:

> "Runny nose with clear snivel and inability to smell foul odors means exactly a vacuity cold condition."

When lung qì is vacuous and cold, yáng qì is unable to perfuse the orifices and distribute liquid, so that it collects in the nose, causing clear snivel that persists for years without recovery.

📖 *Zhèng Zhì Yào Jué* ("Essential Rhymes for Patterns and Treatment"), "Collecting Rheum and Deep-Lying Phlegm"

> "All panting, cough, retching, diarrhea, heart clamor, fearful throbbing, fright palpitations, aversion to cold and heat effusion with pain and swelling, glomus, occlusion, congestion, and block, possibly with gurgling sounds in the chest and rib-side or with an ice-cold area in the back or heart, is caused by phlegm-rheum."

This quotation describes how phlegm-rheum collecting in the chest, diaphragm, heart, and lung prevents heart-lung yáng qì from diffusing and moving, causing numerous symptoms such as cough and panting, heart palpitations, and cold in the back.

📖 *Shèng Jì Zǒng Lù* ("Sages' Salvation Records"), "Section on the Lung Viscus"

> "It is said that puffy swelling of lung qì, of the face and eyes, and of the limbs manifests in cough with distention and fullness, similar to the appearance of water qì. The lung governs qì, and qì is yáng. Since yáng in the body is light and vacuous, it can be turned around by cold and effused to the outside. Dissipating into the skin, the result is qì counterflow and puffy swelling."

The lung is the upper source of water. When the lung's yáng qì is insufficient, it is unable to regulate the waterways, and fluid spills into the skin, to create water swelling.

📖 *Gū Sòng Yuán Yī Jìng* ("Gū Sòng-Yuán's Mirror of Medicine"), "Expounding Pathoconditions and Formulas; Phlegm-Rheum"

> "Cough and counterflow with propped breathing, shortness of breath with inability to lie down, and generalized swelling is called propping rheum."

Propping rheum means that rheum is collecting in the chest and lung. When lung yáng is vacuous and therefore unable to distribute fluids, they transmute into phlegm-rheum, influence the diffusion and downbearing of lung qì, and cause symptoms like cough and panting with copious phlegm, and propped breathing with inability to lie down.

📖 *Bù Jū Jí* ("The Variability Collection"), "Synopsis of Phlegm Patterns"

> "The arrival of phlegm is primarily caused by the lung. Furthermore, since persons with vacuity detriment invariably suffer from a vacuity of lung qì, this prevents lung qì from distributing water and essence throughout the body, so that turbidity congeals and gathers."

This quotation discusses the close link between the formation of phlegm-rheum and lung qì vacuity. In this context, debilitation of the lung's yáng qì disorders the lung's diffusion and depurative downbearing and prevents the dissipation, distribution, and transformation of the fluids. This is the main reason why phlegm-rheum forms and congeals in the lung.

文献评述

《千金要方•肺虚实•肺虚冷》曰: "肺寒损伤，气嗽及涕唾鼻塞。" 寒邪伤肺，损伤肺阳，肺气不通而鼻塞；津液凝滞而流涕唾。

《圣济总录•肺脏门》曰: "论曰肺藏虚弱，为风邪所伤，则清冷之气上攻，而鼻流清涕。盖肺开窍于鼻，在液为涕也。" 肺阳虚，不能布津，转变为涕，则清涕不断。

《辨证录•鼻渊》曰："人有鼻流清涕，经年不愈，是肺气虚寒。"又说："但流清涕而不腥臭，正虚寒之病也。"肺气虚寒，阳气不能宣窍布津，停留鼻窍，故清涕年久不愈。

《证治要诀•停饮伏痰》曰："凡为喘，咳，呕，泄，心嘈，怔忡，惊悸、寒热痛肿，痞膈壅闭，或胸胁间沥沥有声，或背心一片如冰冷，皆痰饮之所致。"论述痰饮停于胸膈心肺，心肺阳气不得宣通，可引起咳喘、心悸、背冷等诸多症状。

《圣济总录•肺脏门》曰："论曰肺气面目四肢浮肿者，其候咳嗽胀满，状如水气。盖肺主气，气为阳，阳体轻虚，为寒所折，攻发于外，散于皮肤，气逆浮肿。"肺为水之上源，肺的阳气不足，不能通调水道，水液泛溢肌肤，而成水肿。

《顾松园医镜•症方发明•痰饮》曰："咳逆倚息，气短不得卧，其形如肿者，曰支饮。"支饮为饮停胸肺，肺阳虚不能输布津液，转变为痰饮，影响肺气宣降，则为咳喘痰多，倚息不卧等症。

《不居集•痰证扼要》曰："痰之来也，多由于肺，而虚损之人肺气未有不虚者，肺气虚则不能水精四布，而浊瘀凝聚也。"论述痰饮的形成，与肺气虚有密切的关系。其中肺的阳气虚衰，宣发肃降失调，水津不得宣散布化，是导致痰饮形成，凝滞于肺的重要原因。

Summary of Lung Cold with Collecting Liquid

1. Lung Cold and Distribution Failure; Liquid Collecting in the Nose
   Clear snivel that runs profusely and incessantly, inability to smell bad or fishy odors, itchy nose, reduced sense of smell.
2. Lung Cold with Collecting Liquid; Transforming into Phlegm-Rheum
   Panting and cough, ejection of clear thin phlegm that is copious and white, the appearance of white froth, drool foaming at the mouth, cough and counterflow with propped breathing and inability to lie down.
3. Qì Failing to Transform Liquid; Liquid Failing to Thrust Out from the Upper Body
   Dryness of the mouth and throat, thirst with a liking for hot drinks, parched skin.
4. Yáng Qì Inside the Chest Unable to Warm the Back
   Aversion to cold in a palm-sized area of the back.
5. Stopped Depurative Downbearing; Spillage of the Fluids
   Water swelling.

肺寒津停
肺寒失布、津停鼻窍——清涕长流不止，不臭而腥，鼻痒，嗅觉减退。
肺寒津停、化生痰饮——咳嗽气喘，吐痰清稀，量多色白，呈泡沫状，口吐涎沫，咳逆倚息不得卧。
气不化津、津不上达——口燥咽干，渴喜热饮，皮肤焦枯。
胸中阳气、不能暖背——背恶寒如掌大。
肃降不行、水液泛溢——水肿。

5.3 Lung Cold with Congealing Blood

The lung assembles the hundred vessels and governs management and regulating. Lung yáng provides warmth and nourishment, promotes movement and assists the heart in moving blood, and safeguards the regular movement of qì and blood. When lung yáng is debilitated, yīn cold becomes internally exuberant, yáng fails to promote movement, the hundred channels contract and tighten, and the blood flow slows down and becomes stagnant. Blood stasis from congealing cold gradually leads to stasis and obstruction of lung blood. Blood stasis in the lung can obstruct lung qì, which results in fullness and oppression in the chest, panting and shortness of breath, and cough and counterflow with propped breathing and inability to lie down. When lung blood is static and obstructed, it cannot be diffused to the head and face, limbs, and skin. The result is a somber facial complexion, green-blue or purple lips and nails, parched hair, dark tongue with stasis macules or stasis speckles, contorted sublingual network vessels, and a rough sunken pulse.

This condition is treated by warming the lung and boosting qì, and by quickening blood and transforming stasis. The recommended formula is *huáng qí guì zhī wǔ wù tāng* (Astragalus and Cinnamon Twig Five Agents Decoction) from the *Jīn Guì Yào Lüe* ("Essential Prescriptions of the Golden Coffer") in combination with *gān cǎo gān jiāng tāng* (Licorice and Dried Ginger Decoction) with additions.

Huáng Qí Guì Zhī Wǔ Wù Tāng 黄耆桂枝五物汤 (Astragalus and Cinnamon Twig Five Agents Decoction)
huáng qí 黄耆 (Astragali Radix, astragalus)
guì zhī 桂枝 (Cinnamomi Ramulus, cinnamon twig)
sháo yào 芍药 (Paeoniae Radix, peony)
shēng jiāng 生姜 (Zingiberis Rhizoma Recens, fresh ginger)
dà zǎo 大枣 (Jujubae Fructus, jujube)

Gān Cǎo Gān Jiāng Tāng 甘草干姜汤
(Licorice and Dried Ginger Decoction)

gān cǎo 甘草 (Glycyrrhizae Radix, licorice)
gān jiāng 干姜 (Zingiberis Rhizoma, dried ginger)
Plus:
chuān xiōng 川芎 (Chuanxiong Rhizoma, chuanxiong)
táo rén 桃仁 (Persicae Semen, peach kernel)
xìng rén 杏仁 (Armeniacae Semen, apricot kernel)
jié gěng 桔梗 (Platycodonis Radix, platycodon)

肺寒血凝

肺朝百脉，主治节，肺阳温养、推动有利助心行血，保证气血正常运行。肺阳虚衰，阴寒内盛，阳失推动，百脉收引，血流缓慢，郁滞难行，寒凝血瘀，渐致肺血瘀阻。肺为血瘀，阻滞肺气，则为胸部满闷、喘息气短、咳逆倚息不得卧；肺血瘀阻，不能布散于头面、四肢、皮肤，则为面色晦暗、唇甲青紫、毛发焦枯、舌暗有瘀斑瘀点、舌下脉络迂曲、脉沉涩等症。治宜温肺益气，活血化瘀。方选《金匮要略》黄芪桂枝五物汤（黄芪、桂枝、芍药、生姜、大枣）合甘草干姜汤，加川芎、桃仁、杏仁、桔梗。

Literature Review of Lung Cold with Congealing Blood

📖 *Yī Biǎn* (“Lancing Stones of Medicine”), “Cough”

> “Panting, fullness, and rapid breathing upon moving indicate distention of the lung. In severe cases, the sternum is elevated, either on the left or on the right, and the person is unable to sleep. This is a disorder caused by phlegm and static blood hampering qì.”

The disease of lung distention is a chronic disease pattern caused by recurring cough and panting. Prolonged cough and panting will invariably damage the lung’s yáng qì. When yáng is vacuous, it fails to promote movement, the blood flow slows down, and lung blood becomes stagnant. Static blood together with phlegm impedes lung qì, which can lead to symptoms like cough, panting, oppression in the chest and rapid breathing, and inability to lie flat.

文献评述

《医碥•咳嗽》曰：“动而喘满气急者，肺胀也。甚则胸骨高昂，或左或右，不能眠，此痰挟瘀血碍气为病。” 肺胀病是反复咳喘而致的慢性病证，久病咳喘必然损伤肺的阳气，阳虚失于推动，血行迟慢，而肺血瘀滞。瘀血挟痰，阻碍肺气，则可引起咳嗽、气喘、胸闷气急，不能平卧等症。

Summary of Lung Cold with Congealing Blood

1. Lung Cold with Congealing Blood; Obstructing Lung Qì
   Fullness and oppression in the chest, panting and shortness of breath, propped breathing with inability to lie down.
2. Lung Blood Stasis and Obstruction; Outward Manifestation of Static Blood
   Somber facial complexion, green-blue or purple lips and nails, parched hair, dark tongue with stasis macules or stasis speckles, contorted sublingual network vessels, rough sunken pulse.

肺寒血凝

肺寒血凝、阻滞肺气——胸部满闷，喘息气短，倚息不卧。

肺血瘀阻、瘀色外现——面色晦暗，唇甲青紫，毛发焦枯，舌暗有瘀斑瘀点，舌下脉络迂曲，脉沉涩。

5.4 Lung Cold with Loss of Restraint

The elimination of urine by the bladder is closely related to steaming qì transformation by kidney yáng. In addition, however, it is also subjected to restraint by the lung's yáng qì. When yáng qì inside the lung is effulgent, diffusion and depurative downbearing move the fluids down into the bladder, and the elimination of urine is normal. However, debilitation of lung yáng and vacuity cold inside the lung causes the lobes of the lung to wither and retract and to lack the strength to contract and retain. Thus, the upper source of water loses its restraint and has no strength to control the urinary bladder. In so-called upper body vacuity with inability to control the lower body, the fluids rush directly into the bladder, which leads to long and frequent voidings of clear urine and in severe cases, to enuresis.

This pathomechanism was first mentioned in the "Treatise on Qì Reversal" in the *Sù Wèn* ("Plain Questions"): "When the heart shifts cold into the lung, the result is lung dispersion. Lung dispersion means passing twice as much fluid as is drunk. It leads to death and cannot be treated." This quotation describes an upper burner dispersion pattern in the context of dispersion-thirst disease: Because lung yáng is vacuous, the upper body fails to control the lower body, which results in profuse urination.

In addition, lung wilting commonly leads to enuresis. For example, the chapter, "Lung Wilting, Lung Welling-Abscess, Cough, and Qì Ascent" in the *Jīn Guì Yào Lüe* ("Essential Prescriptions of the Golden Coffer") explains:

> "In lung wilting, a patient with drool foaming at the mouth but no cough will not be thirsty, but invariably suffer from enuresis and frequent urination. The reason for this is that vacuity in the upper body causes inability to control the lower body. This means cold inside the lung."

This quotation provides powerful proof that lung cold and failure of the upper body to control the lower body leads to copious urine and enuresis.

This condition is treated by warming the lung and dissipating cold, and by boosting qì and securing containment. The recommended formula is *gān cǎo gān jiāng tāng* (Licorice and Dried Ginger Decoction) from the *Jīn Guì Yào Lüe* ("Essential Prescriptions of the Golden Coffer") with additions (see below). As Zhāng Jǐng-Yuè explained:

> "In spite of the fact that urine is disinhibited by the kidney, the kidney is linked to the lung above, and if lung qì is disabled, kidney water eventually cannot be contained. Therefore, to treat water you must first treat qì, and to treat the kidney you must first treat the lung (*Jǐng Yuè Quán Shū* ("Jǐng-Yuè's Complete Compendium"), "Enuresis")."

Gān Cǎo Gān Jiāng Tāng 甘草干姜汤 (Licorice and Dried Ginger Decoction)
gān cǎo 甘草 (Glycyrrhizae Radix, licorice)
gān jiāng 干姜 (Zingiberis Rhizoma, dried ginger)
Plus:
rén shēn 人参 (Ginseng Radix, ginseng)
huáng qí 黄芪 (Astragali Radix, astragalus)
guì zhī 桂枝 (Cinnamomi Ramulus, cinnamon twig)
fù zǐ 附子 (Aconiti Radix Lateralis Praeparata, processed aconite)

肺寒失制

膀胱的排尿，与肾阳的蒸腾气化有密切的关系，但亦受到肺中阳气的制约。肺中阳气旺盛，宣发肃降水液下行膀胱，尿液得以正常排泄。肺阳虚衰，肺中虚冷，肺叶萎缩，无力收摄，水之上源失制，无力制约膀胱，所谓上虚不能制下，水液直趋膀胱，而致小便清长、频数，甚至遗尿。早在《素问•气厥论》中提到："心移寒于肺则肺消，肺消者饮一溲二，死不治。"此乃消渴病中之上消证，因肺阳虚，上不制下而引起小便量多。此外，肺痿常致小便遗尿。如《金匮要略•肺痿肺痈咳嗽上气篇》说："肺痿，吐涎沫而不咳者，其人不渴，必遗尿，小便数，所以然者，以上虚不能制下故也，此为肺中冷。”是对肺寒上不制下而致尿多、遗尿的有力论证。治宜温肺散寒，益气固摄。方选《金匮要略》甘草干姜汤加人参、黄芪、桂枝、附子。正如张景岳所说：“小水虽利于肾，而肾上连肺，若肺气无权，则肾水终不能摄，故治水者必先治气，治肾者必先治肺。”（《景岳全书•遗溺》）

Literature Review of Lung Cold with Loss of Restraint

📖 *Shèng Jì Zǒng Lù* (“Sages’ Salvation Records”), “Section on the Lung Viscus; Lung Wilting and Frequent Urination”

> “The *Nèi Jīng* (“The Inner Canon”) states that ‘the true qì of the viscera is stored high up in the lung.’ It also states that ‘despoliation of true qì results in vacuity.’ In the current context, cold inside the lung results in an insufficiency of the lung’s true qì, which in turn results in upper body vacuity for such a person. In vacuity, there is nothing that can control the lower body; thus there is lung wilting in the upper body and frequent urination in the lower body, as well as drool foaming at the mouth and desire to cough but no cough. All these are its symptoms.”

This quotation describes how lung qì vacuity cold and upper body vacuity and inability to control the lower body mean loss of bladder retention, and lead to frequent urination.

文献评述

《圣济总录•肺脏门•肺痿小便数》曰：“论曰内经曰：藏真高于肺。又曰：真气夺则虚。今肺中冷，则肺之真气不足，则其人上虚矣。虚则无以制下，故上为肺痿，下为小便数，以至吐涎沫而欲咳不能者，皆其证也。”论述肺气虚寒，上虚不能制下，膀胱失约，而致小便频数。

Summary of Lung Cold with Loss of Restraint
Long frequent voidings of clear urine, in severe cases enuresis.
肺寒失制
小便清长，频数，甚至遗尿。

When lung yáng vacuity progresses further, it can lead to lung-heart yáng vacuity, lung-spleen yáng vacuity, or lung-kidney yáng vacuity.

5.4.1 Lung-Heart Yáng Vacuity

The heart and the lung both live in the upper burner and lung qì vacuity can also influence heart qì vacuity. If lung yáng is debilitated and fails to warm and move heart blood adequately, this can lead to impaired nourishment to heart yáng and the pathomechanism of lung-heart yáng vacuity. In addition to cough and shortness of breath, fear of cold and cold limbs, you will also observe symptoms like heart palpitations and fearful throbbing, reduced urination and swollen limbs, a somber facial complexion, and green-blue or purple lips and nails. This condition is treated by supplementing and boosting heart and lung yáng. The recommended formula is *gān cǎo gān jiāng tāng* (Licorice and Dried Ginger Decoction) from the *Jīn Guì Yào Lüè* ("Essential Prescriptions of the Golden Coffer") in combination with *bǎo yuán tāng* (Origin-Preserving Decoction) from the *Jǐng Yuè Quán Shū* ("Jǐng-Yuè's Complete Compendium").

Gān Cǎo Gān Jiāng Tāng 甘草干姜汤 (Licorice and Dried Ginger Decoction)
gān cǎo 甘草 (Glycyrrhizae Radix, licorice) *gān jiāng* 干姜 (Zingiberis Rhizoma, dried ginger)

Bǎo Yuán Tāng 保元汤 (Origin-Preserving Decoction)
rén shēn 人参 (Ginseng Radix, ginseng) *huáng qí* 黄芪 (Astragali Radix, astragalus) *guì zhī* 桂枝 (Cinnamomi Ramulus, cinnamon twig) *gān cǎo* 甘草 (Glycyrrhizae Radix, licorice)

Lung-Spleen Yáng Vacuity

The lung belongs to metal and the spleen to earth. When lung yáng is debilitated, the lung's diffusion and downbearing break down and phlegm-rheum collects internally. Since the child can steal the mother's qì, lung yáng can damage spleen yáng, resulting in the pathomechanism of lung-spleen yáng vacuity. In addition to symptoms of lung yáng vacuity, you will also see torpid intake and reduced eating, abdominal distention and sloppy stool, and copious clear-white thin phlegm. This condition is treated by supplementing and boosting lung and spleen yáng. The recommended formula is *lǐ zhōng tāng* (Center-Rectifying Decoction) from the *Shāng Hán Lùn* ("On Cold Damage") with the addition of *huáng qí* (Astragali Radix), *zǐ wǎn* (Asteris Radix), and *kuǎn dōng huā* (Farfarae Flos).

Lǐ Zhōng Tāng 理中汤 (Center-Rectifying Decoction)
rén shēn 人参 (Ginseng Radix, ginseng) *bái zhú* 白术 (Atractylodis Macrocephalae Rhizoma, white atractylodes) *gān cǎo* 甘草 (Glycyrrhizae Radix, licorice) *gān jiāng* 干姜 (Zingiberis Rhizoma, dried ginger)

Lung-Kidney Yáng Vacuity

The lung is metal, and kidney is water. When lung yáng is debilitated, the disease of the mother can affect the child. Consequently, failure to warm and nourish kidney-water can lead to kidney yáng insufficiency and the pathomechanism of lung-kidney yáng vacuity. Common symptoms of this condition are aversion to cold and cold limbs, enduring cough and panting, exhalation more than inhalation, which is aggravated by movement, and cold aching lumbus and knees. This condition is treated by supplementing and boosting lung and kidney yáng. The recommended formula is *shèn qì wán* (Kidney Qì Pill) from the *Jīn Guì Yào Lüè* ("Essential Prescriptions of the Golden Coffer") or *dà bǔ yuán jiān* (Major Origin-Supplementing Brew) from the *Jǐng Yuè Quán Shū* ("Jǐng-Yuè's Complete Compendium").

Shèn Qì Wán 肾气丸 (Kidney Qì Pill)
shú dì huáng 熟地黄 (Rehmanniae Radix Praeparata, cooked rehmannia) *shān yào* 山药 (Dioscoreae Rhizoma, dioscorea) *shān zhū yú* 山茱萸 (Corni Fructus, cornus) *zé xiè* 泽泻 (Alismatis Rhizoma, alisma) *mǔ dān pí* 牡丹皮 (Moutan Cortex, moutan) *fú líng* 茯苓 (Poria, poria) *guì zhī* 桂枝 (Cinnamomi Ramulus, cinnamon twig) *fù zǐ* 附子 (Aconiti Radix Lateralis Praeparata, processed aconite)

Dà Bǔ Yuán Jiān 大补元煎 (Major Origin-Supplementing Brew)
rén shēn 人参 (Ginseng Radix, ginseng) *dù zhòng* 杜仲 (Eucommiae Cortex, eucommia) *shú dì huáng* 熟地黄 (Rehmanniae Radix Praeparata, cooked rehmannia) *shān yào* 山药 (Dioscoreae Rhizoma, dioscorea) *dāng guī* 当归 (Angelicae Sinensis Radix, Chinese angelica) *shān zhū yú* 山茱萸 (Corni Fructus, cornus) *gǒu qǐ zǐ* 枸杞子 (Lycii Fructus, lycium)

肺阳虚进一步发展，可兼肺心阳虚，肺脾阳虚，肺肾阳虚等症。

肺心阳虚: 心肺同居上焦，肺气虚可影响心气虚，若肺阳虚衰，不足以温运心血，亦可致心阳失养，引起肺心阳虚的病机。除见咳嗽气短，畏寒肢冷外，还见心悸怔忡、尿少肢肿、面色晦暗、唇甲青紫等症。治宜补益心肺之阳。方选《金匮要略》甘草干姜汤合《景岳全书》保元汤。

肺脾阳虚: 肺金脾土，肺阳虚衰，肺失宣降，痰饮内停，子盗母气，损伤脾阳，进而引起肺脾阳虚的病机。除见肺阳虚的表现外，兼见纳呆食少、腹胀便溏、痰多色白清稀等症。治宜补益肺脾之阳。方选《伤寒论》理中汤加黄芪、紫菀、冬花。

肺肾阳虚: 肺金肾水，肺阳虚衰，母病及子，不能温养肾水，可致肾阳不足，引起肺肾阳虚的病机。常见畏寒肢冷、久病咳喘、呼多吸少、动则尤甚、腰膝酸冷等症。治宜补益肺肾之阳。方选《金匮要略》肾气丸，或《景岳全书》大补元煎（人参、杜仲、熟地、山药、当归、山茱萸、枸杞）。

Chapter Six

Lung Yīn Vacuity

Depletion of the lung's yīn humor and failure to moisten can cause a series of pathomechanical changes. The chapter, "Jade Slip" in the *Líng Shū* ("The Magic Pivot") states: "[Lung yīn vacuity is characterized by cough, extreme emaciation, generalized heat effusion, and a small pulse that is racing." Further, the chapter, "Jade Swivel Treatise on True Visceral Pulses" in the *Sù Wèn* ("Plain Questions") states:

> "[Yīn vacuity manifests with] major bone desiccation, wasting and sagging of the major masses of flesh, qì fullness in the chest, panting and absence of bowel movements, internal pain stretching to the shoulder and nape, generalized heat effusion, and shedding of flesh and loss of bulk."

These are the earliest records in the *Nèi Jīng* ("The Inner Canon") to mention yīn vacuity.

In the chapter, "Pulse Symptoms and Treatments of Lung Wilting, Pulmonary Welling-Abscess, Cough, and Qì Ascent" in the *Jīn Guì Yào Lüe* ("Essential Prescriptions of the Golden Coffer"), the Hàn dynasty author Zhāng Zhòng-Jǐng stated:

> "Heat in the upper burner is due to cough causing lung wilting. How does one contract the disease of lung wilting? The teacher said: It is caused by severe fluid collapse, either from sweating, from vomiting, from dispersion-thirst with frequent uninhibited urination, or from difficult defecation that has turned into diarrhea from ingesting disinhibiting medicinals."

This quotation points out that excessive sweating, vomiting, or diarrhea can greatly damage yīn humor and thereby easily turn into lung wilting. However, the *Nèi Jīng, Shāng Hán Zá Bìng Lùn,* and *Zhū Bìng Yuán Hòu Lùn* all discuss the pathomechanism of yīn vacuity only in general terms and focus much more on the other organs, such as the kidney, liver, and stomach.

By the Sòng period, authors were finally discussing the pathomechanism of lung repletion heat resulting from causes like yáng heat exuberance or dryness-heat damaging liquid, more frequently and at least mentioned lung yīn vacuity. In the *Xiǎo Ér Yào Zhèng Zhí Jué* ("Key to Diagnosis and Treatment of Children's Diseases"), Qián Yǐ introduced the disease pattern of "infantile lung vacuity causing rough breathing and hasty panting." The formula for *ē jiāo sǎn* (Ass Hide Glue Powder), also called *bǔ fèi tāng* (Lung-Supplementing Decoction), which was established by him as the treatment for "lung yīn vacuity detriment," has been recognized by most doctors in later generations. Unfortunately, he still did not directly mention the pathomechanism of lung yīn vacuity. Subsequently, the great master of the yīn-supplementing school Zhū Dān-Xī stated: "Yáng is often in superabundance, and yīn is often insufficient." Together with the ideas in Zhāng Jǐng-Yuè's "Treatise on True Yīn," these authors emphasized that kidney yīn depletion coud invade lung yīn, though still without directly discussing damage to lung yīn.

The chapter titled "Yīn Vacuity Conditions are Associated with the Lung" in the *Lǐ Xū Yuán Jiàn* ("The Original Mirror of Rectifying Vacuity") explained:

> "As regards yīn vacuity developing into consumption being associated with the lung, there are a number of different kinds… but all these can be treated completely by governing the lung. The reason for this is that the condition of yīn vacuity consumption, while also called 'five taxations and seven damages,' can be summed up as the lung is the supreme principle."

The famous thesis in this text, that "conditions of yīn vacuity are tied to the lung," is the earliest description of the pathomechanism of lung yīn vacuity.

Afterwards, the rise of the warm disease school in the Qīng dynasty added further depth to the recognition of the pathomechanism of lung yīn vacuity. When scanning the ancient records, they mostly discuss lung yīn vacuity in conjunction with yīn vacuity in the other organs, such as lung-kidney yīn vacuity or lung-stomach yīn vacuity. Records that mention lung yīn vacuity separately are extremely rare. During the process of compiling national advanced teaching materials for Chinese medicine after the founding of the PRC in 1949, the pathomechanism of lung yīn vacuity has finally been formally recognized and completely developed.

Disease causes for lung yīn vacuity include the following: External contraction of the six excesses, especially the evil of warm-heat dryness; an invasion of consumption worms; dietary irregularities, habitual fondness for tobacco and liquor or acrid, hot, and drying foods; disharmony between the five viscera and blazing of internal fire; insufficiency of earlier heaven and weak health in old age; enduring or severe disease, and lack of or inappropriate treatment; or excessive sexual taxation that desiccates kidney water and prevents water from engendering metal. The pathomechanism of lung yīn vacuity can be differentiated into yīn vacuity with loss of nourishment, yīn vacuity with loss of restraint, and yīn vacuity with flaming fire.

肺阴虚

肺之阴津亏损，失于滋润，可引起一系列病机变化。

《灵枢•玉版》曰:“咳，脱形，身热、脉小以疾。”《素问•玉机真脏论》曰:“大骨枯槁，大肉陷下，胸中气满，喘息不便，内痛引肩项，身热，脱肉破䐃。”这是《内经》中最早涉及阴虚的记载。汉代张仲景《金匮要略•肺痿肺痈咳嗽上气病脉证治》云:“热在上焦者因咳为肺痿。肺痿之病，从何得之？师曰: 或从汗出，或从呕吐，或从消渴，小便利数，或从便难，又被快药下利，重亡津液，故得之。”指出汗吐下太过，阴液大伤，易形成肺痿。但是《内经》、《伤寒杂病论》、《诸病源候论》都是综合论述阴虚的病机，尤多涉及肾、肝、胃等其它脏腑。直到宋代之前，对肺的阳热亢盛，燥热伤津等肺实热的病机讨论较多，极少提到肺的阴虚。钱乙《小儿药证直诀》根据“小儿肺虚，气粗喘促”的病证，制定阿胶散（又名补肺汤）是后世诸多医家所公认的治疗“肺阴虚损”的方剂，惜未能正式提出肺阴虚的病机。其后著名补阴派大师朱丹溪提出:“阳常有余，阴常不足”，以及张景岳的“真阴论”思想，都是强调肾阴亏损，上犯于肺阴，未直接论及肺阴的损伤。《理虚元鉴•阴虚之症统于肺》说:“就阴虚成痨之统于肺者而言，均有数种。…凡此种种，悉宰于肺治。所以然者，阴虚痨症，虽有五劳七伤之异名，而要之以肺为极则。”从而提出“阴虚之症统于肺”的著明论点，这是对肺阴虚病机的最早论述。在此之后，清代温病学派的兴起，对肺阴虚病机的认识更加深入。纵观古代文献，大多将肺阴虚与其它脏腑阴虚的病机相提并论，如肺肾阴虚、肺胃阴虚等等，单独提肺阴虚的甚少。直到解放以后编写全国高等中医教材时，肺阴虚的病机才正式得以确认，发展完善。肺阴虚的病因包括外感六淫，特别是温热燥邪；或痨虫侵袭；或饮食不节，素嗜烟酒、辛热燥辣食物；或五脏失和，内火燔灼；或先天不足，老年体弱；或久病重病，失治误治；或房劳太过，肾水枯竭，水不生金，均可导致。肺阴虚的病机可分为阴虚失养，阴虚失制，阴虚火炎等几个方面。

6.1 Yīn Vacuity with Loss of Nourishment

Lung yīn is the most important material base for nourishing the lung and for maintaining its physiological functions. When lung yīn is depleted, it fails to be nourished, which can lead to a variety of functional irregularities in the lung. If the diffusing and depurative downbearing functions are deprived of moistening by lung yīn, depuration cannot take place and lung qì will ascend counterflow, manifesting in qì counterflow panting and cough. If there is a lack of fluids inside the lung, they cannot be converted into phlegm, which results in symptoms like dry cough without phlegm or with scanty sticky phlegm that is not easily expectorated, clear high coughing sound, and severe cough.

The "Treatise on Dry Cough" in the *Lǐ Xū Yuán Jiàn* ("The Original Mirror of Rectifying Vacuity") states: "Dry cough refers to a sound but no phlegm. This condition is caused by an insufficiency of essence blood, water failing to help fire, fire qì flaming upward, and true yīn being scorched. Fire in the lung seeps out, causing dryness and cough."

The chapter, "The Origin and Development of Cough, Wheezing, and Panting" in the *Zá Bìng Yuán Liú Xī Zhú* ("Incisive Light on the Source of Miscellaneous Disease") also explains:

> "Ten: Dry cough means that there are no fluids inside the lung. The pulse of such a person is fine and rough… Mild cases present with continuous coughing that after more than ten coughs finally produces phlegm; severe cases present with profuse coughing but no ejection of phlegm. Therefore it constitutes dry cough, which is extremely difficult to treat."

Both these quotations illustrate the important pathomechanism by which lung yīn failing to enrich and insufficiency of fluids leads to dry cough.

This condition is treated by enriching yīn and moistening the lung, and by transforming phlegm and suppressing cough. The recommended formula is *shā shēn mài dōng tāng* (Adenophora/glehnia and Ophiopogon Decoction) from the *Wēn Bìng Tiáo Bian* ("Systematized Identification of Warm Diseases").

Shā Shēn Mài Dōng Tāng 沙参麦冬汤 (Adenophora/glehnia and Ophiopogon Decoction)
shā shēn 沙参 (Adenophorae seu Glehniae Radix, adenophora/glehnia)
mài mén dōng 麦门冬(Ophiopogonis Radix, ophiopogon)
sāng yè 桑叶 (Mori Folium, mulberry leaf)
yù zhú 玉竹 (Polygonati Odorati Rhizoma, Solomon's seal)
bái biǎn dòu 白扁豆 (Lablab Semen Album, lablab)
tiān huā fěn 天花粉 (Trichosanthis Radix, trichosanthes root)
gān cǎo 甘草 (Glycyrrhizae Radix, licorice)

If insufficiency of lung yīn prevents the fluids from being distributed all over the body, nourishment to the formal body, the flesh, the skin and body hair, and the stool and urine is impaired. This can lead to symptoms like emaciation, dry mouth, nose, and throat, a haggard complexion, and parched skin and body hair. As the chapter, "Dryness Damage" in the *Yī Biǎn* ("Lancing Stones of Medicine") states:

> "In blood collapse or liquid collapse, the kidney is vacuous and fire exuberant. The various causes of this condition are associated with man-made factors. Outwardly, it manifests in chapped, raw, and dry skin; in the upper body, in parched nose and throat; in the lower body, in desiccated stool and urine; in the extremities, in wilting and lack of strength; and in the pulse, in roughness, stagnation, vacuity, and debilitation. Treat this condition with sweet, cold, and moistening preparations, and clear the lung to enrich the source of water, in the hope that by making the blood and yīn full you can moisturize the hundred bones."

While this quotation discusses dryness damage, the treatment method with sweet, cold, and moistening preparations to clear the lung and thereby enrich the source of water offers insights into the pathomechanism of lung yīn depletion and loss of nourishment in the whole body.

This condition is treated by enriching yīn and clearing heat, and by engendering liquid and moistening the lung. The recommended formula is *qīng zào jiù fèi tāng* (Dryness-Clearing Lung-Rescuing Decoction) from the *Yī Mén Fǎ Lǜ* ("Axioms of Medicine").

Qīng Zào Jiù Fèi Tāng 清燥救肺汤 (Dryness-Clearing Lung-Rescuing Decoction)
sāng yè 桑叶 (Mori Folium, mulberry leaf)
shí gāo 石膏 (Gypsum Fibrosum, gypsum)
rén shēn 人参 (Ginseng Radix, ginseng)
mài mén dōng 麦门冬 (Ophiopogonis Radix, ophiopogon)
xìng rén 杏仁 (Armeniacae Semen, apricot kernel)
pí pá yè 枇杷叶 (Eriobotryae Folium, loquat leaf)
hēi zhī má 黑脂麻 (Sesami Semen Nigrum, black sesame)
ē jiāo 阿胶 (Asini Corii Colla, ass hide glue)
gān cǎo 甘草 (Glycyrrhizae Radix, licorice)

The lung is the delicate viscus; the lobes of the lung are tender. When lung yīn is depleted and thus unable to enrich the lobes of the lung, they dry out, manifesting as lung wilting. Commonly observed symptoms include stretched mouth with shortness of breath and cough with spitting of foamy turbid spittle and drool. This is directly explained in the chapter, "Lung Wilting, Lung Welling-Abscess, Cough, and Qì Ascent" in the *Jīn Guì Yào Lüe* ("Essential Prescriptions of the Golden Coffer"):

> "When there is heat in the upper burner, cough causes lung wilting. How does one contract lung wilting disease? The teacher said: It is caused by severe fluid collapse from sweating, from vomiting, from dispersion-thirst with disinhibited and frequent urination, or from difficult defecation that has turned into diarrhea due to taking disinhibiting medicinals."

This statement explains that yīn humor depletion is an important cause of lung wilting.

When the lobes of the lung wither, depuration stops and the fluids are not distributed but transform into foamy drool. Thus we observe drool foaming at the mouth in spite of the fact that lung yīn is deficient. The chapter, "Pulmonary Welling-Abscess and Wilting" in the *Yī Mén Fǎ Lǜ* ("Axioms of Medicine") explains:

> "Lung wilting, being cumulative and gradual, will not end in one day, and cold and heat will not stop with only one extreme. It is always caused by a failure to move the fluids inside the stomach to the lung, so that the lung is deprived of nourishment and becomes dry. This is how lung wilting arises… This means merely that the fluids that are supplied to the upper body are consumed on branch roads. As a result, lung fire intensifies every day, lung heat deepens every day, the small ducts inside the lung become more asphyxiated every day, the sound of cough gradually fails to be effused, and the fat layers inside the chest dry out. The result is cough with phlegm that is difficult to raise and expel, with frequent fierce activity. Breathing will be characterized by panting and rale that develops into continuously-sounding surges before the phlegm begins to respond (i.e. be expectorated)."

This quotation further illustrates the pathomechanism by which lung dryness and damaged liquid impairs moistening and leads to lung wilting.

This condition is treated by enriching yīn and clearing and moistening lung heat. The recommended formula is *mài mén dōng tāng* (Ophiopogon Decoction) from the *Jīn Guì Yào Lüe* ("Essential Prescriptions of the Golden Coffer") with additions.

Mài Mén Dōng Tāng 麦门冬汤 (Ophiopogon Decoction)
mài mén dōng 麦门冬 (Ophiopogonis Radix, ophiopogon)
bàn xià 半夏 (Pinelliae Rhizoma, pinellia)
rén shēn 人参 (Ginseng Radix, ginseng)
gēng mǐ 粳米 (Oryzae Semen, non-glutinous rice)
gān cǎo 甘草 (Glycyrrhizae Radix, licorice)
Plus:
dàn zhú yè 淡竹叶 (Lophatheri Herba, lophatherum)
shí gāo 石膏(Gypsum Fibrosum, gypsum)

阴虚失滋

肺阴是滋养肺脏，维持肺的生理功能活动的重要物质基础。肺阴亏虚，失于滋养，可引起肺的多种功能失调。宣发肃降功能缺乏肺阴的滋润，清肃之令不行，肺气上逆，发为咳喘气逆。肺中津液缺乏，不能转化为痰，故见干咳无痰、或痰少而粘、不易咯出、咳声清高、咳嗽剧烈等症。如《理虚元鉴•干咳嗽论》云："干咳者，有声无痰，病因精血不足，水不济火，火气上炎，真阴燔灼，肺脏火渗涩而咳也。"《杂病源流犀烛•咳嗽哮喘源流》亦说："十曰干嗽，肺中无津液也，其脉细涩。…轻则连咳数十声，方有痰出，重则多咳亦不吐痰，故为干咳嗽，极难治。"均阐明肺阴失滋，津少不足，是引起干咳的重要病机。治宜滋阴润肺，化痰止咳。方选《温病条辨》沙参麦冬汤（沙参、麦冬、桑叶、玉竹、扁豆、花粉、甘草）；若肺阴不足，津液不能敷布全身，形体、肌肉、皮毛、二便失养，可致形体消瘦、口鼻咽喉干燥、面色憔悴、皮毛焦枯等症。如《医碥•伤燥》曰："若亡血亡津，肾虚火盛，致此多端，则又属于人事矣。在外则皮肤皴揭枯涩，在上则鼻咽焦干，在下则二便涸涩，在手足则痿弱无力，在脉则涩滞虚衰。治以甘寒润剂，清肺以滋水源，庶几血充阴满，泽及百骸。"此处虽言伤燥，但从治法甘寒润剂，清肺以滋水源，可悟出肺阴亏虚，全身失滋的病机。治宜滋阴清热、生津润肺。方选《医门法律》清燥救肺汤（桑叶、石膏、人参、麦冬、杏仁、枇杷叶、胡麻仁、阿胶、甘草）；肺为娇脏，肺叶娇嫩，肺阴亏虚，不能滋养肺叶，肺叶干枯，发为肺痿，常见张口短气、咳吐浊唾涎沫等症。正如《金匮要略•肺痿肺痈咳嗽上气篇》所说："热在上焦者，因咳为肺痿，肺痿从何得之？师曰：或从汗出，或从呕吐，或从消渴小便利数，或从便难，又被快药下利，重亡津液，故得之。"说明阴液亏损是产生肺痿的主要原因。肺叶枯萎，清肃不行，水津不布，化为涎沫，故虽肺阴缺乏而反见呕吐涎沫。《医门法律•肺痈肺痿门》说："肺痿者，其积渐已非一日，其寒热不止一端，总由胃中津液不输于肺，肺失所养，转枯转燥，然后成之。…只此上供之津液，坐耗歧途。于是肺火日炽，肺热日深，肺中小管日窒，咳声以渐不扬，胸中脂膜日干，咳痰难于上出，行动数武，气即喘鸣，冲击连声，痰始一应。"亦进一步阐明肺燥津伤，失于滋润而致肺痿的病机。治宜滋阴清润肺热。方选《金匮要略》麦门冬汤（麦冬、半夏、人参、粳米、甘草）加竹叶、石膏。

Literature Review of Yīn Vacuity with Failure to Enrich

🕮 *Zhāng Shì Yī Tōng* ("Zhang's Clear View of Medicine"), "Cough"

"Yīn vacuity and taxation cough results in a timid and dry voice, first tense and then relaxed, possibly aggravated in the morning or in the evening, and in clear phlegm, shortage of qì, and panting breath."

This quotation describes the pathomechanism by which yīn vacuity, failure of the lung to moisten and depurate, and counterflow ascent of lung qì result in cough with shortage of qì and panting.

🕮 *Lín Zhèng Zhǐ Nán Yī Àn* ("A Clinical Guide with Case Histories"), "Lung Wilting"

"The condition of lung wilting is generally ascribed to dried fluids and is mostly caused by sweating damaging right qì. The Chinese character for the pathocondition of wilting is related to the character for the natural phenomenon of wilting. The word "wilting" (痿) as a pathocondition comes from "wilting" of plants (萎). Just like the wilting of plants and their loss of luxuriance, the disease is caused by a collapse of liquid and exhaustion of qì.

Regarding the cause of wilting, there are a variety of aspects to consider. The *Jīn Guì Yào Lüe* ("Essential Prescriptions of the Golden Coffer") states that lung heat, dryness, and wilting is caused by severe fluid collapse, either from sweating, from vomiting, from dispersion-thirst with frequent uninhibited urination, or from difficult defecation that has turned into diarrhea due to taking disinhibiting medicinals. Lung heat, dryness, and wilting mean that depuration is not carried out and that the distribution of water and essence throughout the body becomes irregular.

Even though spleen qì disperses the fluids to the upper body and back to the lung, the lung is neither able to moisten its own dryness nor to sprinkle the six bowels inside and transport liquid to the skin and body hair on the outside. Its fluids remain inside the chest and when they are subjected to heat, they boil and transform into foamy drool. When this invades the lung, it causes cough and incessant spitting. The dryness comes from dryness and the spitting from spittle, and the more spittle there is, the more dryness results. This is how wilting disease develops."

This quotation describes the pathomechanism by which damage to the liquids, dried lobes of the lung, and impaired depuration form lung wilting with unproductive cough or cough and spitting of foamy drool.

文献评述

《张氏医通•咳嗽》曰: “阴虚劳嗽则声怯而槁，先急后缓，或早甚，或暮甚，清痰少气而喘气也。”论述阴虚，肺失滋润清肃，肺气上逆，引起咳嗽少气而喘的病机。

《临证指南医案•肺痿》曰: “肺痿一症，概属津枯液燥，多由汗下伤正所致。夫痿者，萎也。如草木之萎而不荣，为津亡而气竭也。然致痿之因，非止一端。《金匮》云: 或从汗出，或从呕吐，或从消渴，小便利数，或从便难，又被快药下之，重亡津液，故令肺热干痿也。肺热干痿，则清肃之令不行，水精四布失度，脾气虽散津液上归于肺，而肺不能自滋其干，亦不能内洒陈于六腑，外输津于皮毛也。其津液留贮胸中，得热煎熬，变为涎沫，侵肺作咳，唾之不已。故干者自干，唾者自唾，愈唾愈干，痿病成矣。”论述津液损伤，肺叶干枯，失于清肃，形成肺痿咳嗽、咳唾涎沫的病机。

Summary of Yīn Vacuity with Loss of Nourishment
1. Stopped Depuration Dry cough without phlegm or with scanty sticky phlegm that is not easily expectorated, high coughing sound, severe coughing. 2. Loss of Enrichment in the Entire Body Emaciation; dry mouth, nose, and throat, haggard complexion, parched skin and body hair. 3. Drying of the Lobes of the Lung Stretched mouth with shortness of breath, cough with spitting of foamy turbid spittle and drool (lung wilting).

阴虚失滋
清肃不行——干咳无痰，或痰少而粘，不易咯出，咳声清高，咳嗽剧烈。 全身失滋——形体消瘦，口鼻咽喉干燥，面色憔悴，皮毛焦枯。 肺叶干枯——张口短气，咳吐浊唾涎沫（肺痿）。

6.2 Yīn Vacuity with Loss of Restraint

The lung governs regulation of the waterways and is the upper source of water. As a result of depurative downbearing by lung qì, the fluids are transported down to the anal and genital orifices, and stool and urine are discharged smoothly. The chapter, "Cough" in the *Xuè Zhèng Lùn* ("On Blood Patterns") contains the following explanation: "The lobes of the lung are plump and moist and droop downward. They restrain and press qì down, causing it to move downward. The fluids follow qì down and also descend. This is how water and liquid are distributed throughout the body." This quotation states that the lung governs management and regulating and is closely related to the elimination of stool and urine.

The lung and the large intestine stand in an exterior-interior relationship. If lung yīn is reduced, the fluids dry up and fail to move down into the large intestine. Having no water to move the boat, conveyance breaks down. This can lead to dry intestines and constipation, a single bowel movement in several days, and difficult defecation.

The chapter, "Dry Bound Stool" in the *Shí Shì Mì Lù* ("Secret Records from the Stone Chamber") explains:

> "People assume that bound stool is caused by severe dryness in the large intestine. Who is aware that it is related to dryness of lung qì? When the lung is dry, depurating qì is unable to move downwards into the large intestine."

Lung dryness is bound to damage yīn, make lung yīn insufficient, stop depuration, and prevent the fluids from descending and enriching the large intestine. The result is constipation and difficult bowel movements.

The "Treatise on Yīn and Yáng, Water and Fire, and Qì and Blood" in the *Xuè Zhèng Lùn* ("On Blood Patterns") further points out: "If water-yīn is insufficient, the fluids are desiccated. Above, this results in wilting and cough since there is no water to relieve the dryness; below, the result is constipation since regulation does not reach the lower body." This quotation also points out that insufficiency of liver yīn and failure to enrich the large intestine is an important pathomechanism for causing constipation.

This condition is treated by enriching yīn and clearing heat, and by moistening the intestines and freeing the stool. The recommended formula is *shā shēn mài dōng tāng* (Adenophora/glehnia and Ophiopogon Decoction) from the *Wēn Bìng Tiáo Bian* ("Systematized Identification of Warm Diseases") in combination with *zēng yè tāng* (Humor-Increasing Decoction) from the same text. An alternate choice is *bǎi hé gù jīn tāng* (Lily Bulb Metal-Securing Decoction) from the *Yī Fāng Jí Jiě* ("Medical Formulas Gathered and Explained") with the addition of *jiù jūn liáng yè* (Pyracanthae Folium).

Shā Shēn Mài Dōng Tāng 沙参麦冬汤 (Adenophora/glehnia and Ophiopogon Decoction)
shā shēn 沙参 (Adenophorae seu Glehniae Radix, adenophora/glehnia)
mài mén dōng 麦门冬 (Ophiopogonis Radix, ophiopogon)
sāng yè 桑叶 (Mori Folium, mulberry leaf)
yù zhú 玉竹 (Polygonati Odorati Rhizoma, Solomon's seal)
bái biǎn dòu 白扁豆 (Lablab Semen Album, lablab)
tiān huā fěn 天花粉 (Trichosanthis Radix, trichosanthes root)
gān cǎo 甘草 (Glycyrrhizae Radix, licorice)

Zēng Yè Tāng 增液汤 (Humor-Increasing Decoction)
xuán shēn 玄参 (Scrophulariae Radix, scrophularia)
mài mén dōng 麦门冬 (Ophiopogonis Radix, ophiopogon)
shēng dì huáng 生地黄 (Rehmanniae Radix, rehmannia)

Bǎi Hé Gù Jīn Tāng 百合固金汤 (Lily Bulb Metal-Securing Decoction)
bǎi hé 百合 (Lilii Bulbus, lily bulb)
mài mén dōng 麦门冬 (Ophiopogonis Radix, ophiopogon)
jié gěng 桔梗 (Platycodonis Radix, platycodon)
bèi mǔ 贝母 (Fritillariae Bulbus, fritillaria)
shú dì huáng 熟地黄 (Rehmanniae Radix Praeparata, cooked rehmannia)
shēng dì huáng 生地黄 (Rehmanniae Radix, rehmannia)
xuán shēn 玄参 (Scrophulariae Radix, scrophularia)
dāng guī 当归 (Angelicae Sinensis Radix, Chinese angelica)
sháo yào 芍药 (Paeoniae Radix, peony)
gān cǎo 甘草 (Glycyrrhizae Radix, licorice)
Plus:
jiù jūn liáng yè 救军粮叶 (Pyracanthae Folium, firethorn leaf)

If shortage of fluids inside the lung has been caused by heat damaging lung yīn, or by an inability of the fluids inside the stomach to move up into the lung, this means that the source of transformation is insufficient, that the formation of urine is reduced, and that qì transformation in the urinary bladder has broken down. This results in shortened rough urination and in severe cases, possibly dribbling urinary block. The chapter, "Pathomechanisms of the Viscera and Bowels" in the *Xuè Zhèng Lùn* ("On Blood Patterns") explains:

> "Ordinarily, there are fluids inside the lung to nourish its metal. Because of this, metal is clear and fire deep-lying. If the fluids are damaged …the source of water is not clear, causing difficult urination, and heat is passed to the large intestine, causing difficult defecation."

This source expounds on the pathomechanism of lung yīn depletion, lack of water in the upper origin, and interruption of flow in the lower origin.

This condition is treated by boosting the stomach and clearing the lung, and by enriching water and unstopping blockage. The recommended formula is *qīng fèi yǐn* (Lung-Clearing Beverage) from the *Zhèng Zhì Huì Bǔ* ("Combined Supplements to Patterns and Treatment") with modifications.

Qīng Fèi Yǐn 泻肺饮 (Lung-Clearing Beverage)
sāng bái pí 桑白皮 (Mori Cortex, mulberry root bark)
huáng qín 黄芩 (Scutellariae Radix, scutellaria)
mài mén dōng 麦门冬 (Ophiopogonis Radix, ophiopogon)
fú líng 茯苓 (Poria, poria)
chē qián zǐ 车前子 (Plantaginis Semen, plantago seed)
mù tōng 木通 (Akebiae Trifoliatae Caulis, trifoliate akebia)
Minus:
zhī zǐ 栀子 (Gardeniae Fructus, gardenia)
Plus:
shān yào 山药 (Dioscoreae Rhizoma, dioscorea)
yù zhú 玉竹 (Polygonati Odorati Rhizoma, Solomon's seal)
shā shēn 沙参 (Adenophorae seu Glehniae Radix, adenophora/glehnia)

If heat damage to lung yīn is so severe that the fluids inside the lung are desiccated and the lung is not moist, depuration stops. Consequently, fluid cannot be distributed to the lower body as normal but spills into the skin, forming water swelling. At the same time, you will observe the symptom of short voidings of scant urine because the fluids fail to be transported down into the urinary bladder. This is exactly the pattern commonly referred to as yīn vacuity water swelling. Its key feature is that it originates in lung-kidney yīn vacuity, which then spreads to affect lung yīn.

When yīn essence is depleted, essence fails to transform qì, yáng functions break down, vacuity heat arises internally, and fluid floods. This is exactly as explained in the "Origin of Swelling and Distention" in the *Zá Bìng Yuán Liú Xī Zhú* ("Incisive Light on the Source of Miscellaneous Disease"): "When kidney water is insufficient, vacuity fire scorches metal, urine is not engendered, and the patient suffers from swelling." When kidney yīn is vacuous, yīn fails to restrain yáng, and vacuity fire flames upward, damaging lung yīn. When lung yīn is vacuous, the lung fails to depurate and downbear. Fluid cannot be moved down, resulting in scant urine, while fluid spilling into the skin causes water swelling.

This condition is treated by enriching the kidney and nourishing the lung, and by disinhibiting water and dispersing swelling. The recommended formula is *liù wèi dì huáng wán* (Six-Ingredient Rehmannia Pill) from the *Xiǎo Ér Yào Zhèng Zhí Jué* ("Key to Diagnosis and Treatment of Children's Diseases") with additions.

Liù Wèi Dì Huáng Wán 六味地黄丸 (Six-Ingredient Rehmannia Pill)

shú dì huáng 熟地黄 (Rehmanniae Radix Praeparata, cooked rehmannia)
shān yào 山药 (Dioscoreae Rhizoma, dioscorea)
fú líng 茯苓 (Poria, poria)
zé xiè 泽泻 (Alismatis Rhizoma, alisma)
mǔ dān pí 牡丹皮 (Moutan Cortex, moutan)
shān zhū yú 山茱萸 (Corni Fructus, cornus)

Plus:

zhū líng 猪苓 (Polyporus, polyporus)
chē qián zǐ 车前子 (Plantaginis Semen, plantago seed)

阴虚失制

肺主通调水道，为水之上源。肺气肃降，津液下输前后二阴，则二便通畅。《血证论•咳嗽》有"肺叶腴润，复垂向下，将气敛抑，使气下行，气下津液随之而降，是以水津四布"之说，即言肺主治节，与二便排泄有密切关系。肺与大肠相表里，若肺阴受损，津液枯少，不能下输大肠，无水行舟，传导失司，可致肠枯便秘，数日一行，排便困难。如《石室秘录•大便燥结》说："大便闭结者，人以为大肠燥甚，谁知是肺气燥乎？肺燥则清肃之气，不能下行于大肠。"肺燥必伤阴，肺阴不足，清肃不行，津液不能下滋大肠，则便秘难行。《血证论•阴阳水火气血论》进一步指出："设水阴不足，津液枯竭，上则痿咳，无水以济之也，下则闭结，制节不达于下也。"均指出肺阴不足，大肠失滋，是导致便秘的重要病机之一。治宜滋阴清热，润肠通便。方选《温病条辨》沙参麦冬汤合《温病条辨》增液汤（玄参、麦冬、生地），亦可用《医方集解》百合固金汤（百合、麦冬、桔梗、贝母、熟地、生地、玄参、当归、芍药、甘草）加酒军；若热伤肺阴，或胃中津液不能上输于肺，肺中津液匮乏，化源不足，小便生成减少，膀胱气化失司，则为小便短涩不畅，甚或癃闭。如《血证论•脏腑病机》说："肺中常有津液养其金，故金清火伏。若津液伤，…水源不清，而小便涩；遗热大肠，而大便难。"这里阐述了肺阴亏损，上源缺水，下源断流的病机。治宜益胃清肺，滋水通闭。方选《证治汇补》清肺饮

（桑白皮、黄芩、麦冬、茯苓、车前仁、木通、栀子）去栀子加山药、玉竹、沙参；若热甚伤阴，肺中津液枯竭而失润，清肃之令不行，水液不能正常向下输布，泛溢肌肤可成水肿，同时因津液不能下输膀胱而兼见小便短少之症。此乃通常所说的阴虚水肿证，主要源于肝肾阴虚，波及肺阴。阴精亏损，精不化气，阳用失司，虚热自生，水液泛溢。诚如《杂病源流犀烛•肿胀源流》所说："肾水不足，虚火灼金，小便不生而患肿。"肾阴虚，阴不制阳，虚火上炎，损伤肺阴，肺阴虚，肺失肃降，水津不能下输而尿少；水津泛溢于肌肤而成水肿。治宜滋肾养肺，利水消肿。方选《小儿药证直诀》六味地黄丸（熟地、山药、茯苓、泽泻、丹皮、山茱萸）加猪苓、车前仁。

Literature Review of Yīn Vacuity with Loss of Restraint

📖 *Zhèng Yīn Mài Zhì* ("Pathoconditions: Causes, Pulses, and Treatments"), "Yīn Vacuity Inhibited Urination"

> "The cause for inhibited urination from yīn vacuity is this: The lung governs the engendering of water, and when lung yīn is insufficient, the source of transformation is disabled, resulting in inhibited urination."

文献评述

《症因脉治•阴虚小便不利》曰："阴虚小便不利之因，肺主生水，肺阴不足，则化源失令而小便不利。"

Summary of Yīn Vacuity with Loss of Restraint
1. Loss of Enrichment in the Large Intestine: Dry intestines and constipation, a single bowel movement in several days, difficult defecation. 2. Reduced Urine: Shortened rough urination, in severe cases possibly dribbling urinary block. 3. Impaired Distribution of Fluid: Scanty urine, water swelling.

阴虚失制
大肠失滋——肠枯便秘，数日一行，排便困难。 小便减少——小便短涩不畅，甚或癃闭。 水津失布——尿少，水肿。

6.3 Yīn Vacuity Flaming Fire

The chapter, "Taxation Consumption" in the *Shòu Shì Bǎo Yuán* ("Prolonging Life and Preserving the Origin") explains:

> "Yīn vacuity stirring fire causes the disease of taxation consumption. It is created by ministerial fire [affecting] lung metal. Damage to a person's essence causes yīn vacuity stirring fire. When such a person's blood is consumed, fire becomes hyperactive, and consequently metal also becomes hyperactive."

This quotation indicates the pathomechanism by which insufficiency of lung yīn, failure of yīn to restrain yáng, and exuberance of yáng qì result in vacuity fire in the lung harassing internally.

When yīn vacuity fire within the lung flames, it condenses fluids to phlegm; phlegm and fire obstruct each other, depuration breaks down, and lung fire surges counterflow. This can lead to incessant cough and counterflow, sticky yellow phlegm, and inhibited coughing and spitting. The chapter, "Coughing of Blood" in the *Xuè Zhèng Lùn* ("On Blood Patterns") states:

> "Severe fire in lung-metal boils fluid into phlegm and damages it. As a result, the lobes of the lung are no longer able to be plump, moist, and drooping. Furthermore, if qì also fumigates the liver and kidney that are located below it, the lobes of the lung are scorched and lifted, so that they are unable to restrain and regulate. Therefore qì moves counterflow, causing cough. The more qì moves counterflow, the more prolonged and incessant the cough becomes."

This condition is treated by enriching yīn and clearing heat, and by moistening the lung and suppressing cough. The recommended formula is *yuè huá wán* (Moonlight Pill) from the *Yī Xué Xīn Wù* ("Medical Insights").

Yuè Huá Wán 月华丸 (Moonlight Pill)
shā shēn 沙参 (Adenophorae seu Glehniae Radix, adenophora/glehnia)
mài mén dōng 门冬 (Ophiopogonis Radix, ophiopogon
tiān dōng 天门冬 (Asparagi Radix, asparagus)
shēng dì huáng 生地黄 (Rehmanniae Radix, rehmannia)
shú dì huáng 熟地黄 (Rehmanniae Radix Praeparata, cooked rehmannia)
ē jiāo 阿胶 (Asini Corii Colla, ass hide glue)
sāng yè 桑叶 (Mori Folium, mulberry leaf)
jú huā 菊花 (Chrysanthemi Flos, chrysanthemum)
chuān bèi mǔ 川贝母 (Fritillariae Cirrhosae Bulbus, Sichuan fritillaria)
bǎi bù 百部 (Stemonae Radix, stemona)
shān yào 山药 (Dioscoreae Rhizoma, dioscorea)
fú líng 茯苓 (Poria, poria)
sān qī 三七 (Notoginseng Radix, notoginseng)
tǎ gān 獭肝 (Lutrae Iecur, otter's liver)

If lung yīn is depleted, lung fire can become progressively more exuberant and the heat can distress the movement of blood and damage the lung's network vessels. This can lead to cough and counterflow with chest pain, phlegm containing blood, and possibly expectoration of bright red blood.

The chapter "Blood Patterns" in "Schema of Miscellaneous Patterns" from the *Jǐng Yuè Quán Shū* ("Jǐng-Yuè's Complete Compendium") provides a direct explanation:

> "All cases of blood disease are without exception caused by water depletion, even though they are differentiated by the five viscera. Water repletion then causes exuberant fire; when fire is exuberant, it torments metal; when metal is diseased, the lung becomes dry. When the lung is dry, the network vessels are damaged, which results in a tendency to cough blood, and humor is desiccated and turns into phlegm."

The chapter "Coughing of Blood" in the *Xuè Zhèng Lùn* ("On Blood Patterns") also explains:

> "The lung is the delicate viscus, and as soon as its fluids are damaged, regardless of whether it is due to external contraction or internal damage, yīn becomes vacuous and fire stirs. The lung is tormented by it, metal loses its ability to carry out depuration, and qì ascends counterflow, causing cough with ejection of phlegm and blood."

When lung vacuity fire flames, it damages the network vessels, and heat forces blood to move. The blood is expelled with cough, thus constituting coughing of blood.

This condition is treated by enriching yīn and clearing heat, and by cooling blood and stanching bleeding. The recommended formula is *bái jī pí pá gāo* (Bletillae and Condensed Loquat Extract) from the *Zhèng Zhì Yào Jué* ("Essential Rhymes for Patterns and Treatment") with additions.

Bái Jī Pí Pá Gāo 白芨枇杷膏 (Bletillae and Condensed Loquat Extract)
shēng dì huáng 生地黄 (Rehmanniae Radix, rehmannia)
ē jiāo 阿胶 (Asini Corii Colla, ass hide glue)
bái jí 白及 (Bletillae Rhizoma, bletilla)
ǒu jié 藕节 (Nelumbinis Rhizomatis Nodus, lotus root node)
pí pá yè 枇杷叶 (Eriobotryae Folium, loquat leaf)
Plus:
cè bǎi yè 侧柏叶 (Platycladi Cacumen, arborvitae leaf)
xiān hè cǎo 仙鹤草 (Agrimoniae Herba, agrimony)
xiǎo jì 小蓟 (Cirsii Herba, field thistle)
xuè yú tàn 血余炭 (Crinis Carbonisatus, charred hair)

In addition, when lung yīn is insufficient, vacuity fire arising internally can lead to generalized vacuity heat patterns, which manifest in generalized low-grade fever, vexing heat in the five hearts, postmeridian tidal heat, and reddening of the cheeks and night sweating. This condition is treated by enriching yīn and clearing heat. The recommended formula is *qīng gǔ sǎn* (Bone-Clearing Powder) from the *Zhèng Zhì Huì Bǔ* ("Combined Supplements to Patterns and Treatment") with the addition of *shēng dì huáng* (Rehmanniae Radix).

Qīng Gǔ Sǎn 清骨散 (Bone-Clearing Powder)
yín chái hú 银柴胡 (Stellariae Radix, stellaria)
hú huáng lián 胡黄连 (Picrorhizae Rhizoma, picrorhiza)
qīng hāo 青蒿 (Artemisiae Annuae Herba, sweet wormwood)
dì gǔ pí 地骨皮 (Lycii Cortex, lycium root bark)
qín jiāo 秦艽 (Gentianae Macrophyllae Radix, large gentian)
biē jiǎ 鳖甲 (Trionycis Carapax, turtle shell)
Plus:
shēng dì huáng 生地黄 (Rehmanniae Radix, rehmannia)

阴虚火炎

《寿世保元•劳瘵》说: "夫阴虚火动，劳瘵之疾，由相火肺金而成也。伤其精则阴虚火动，耗其血则火亢而金亢。" 指出肺阴不足，阴不制阳，阳气亢盛，则为肺脏虚火内扰的病机。肺中阴虚火炎，炼液为痰，痰火交阻，清肃失司，肺火冲逆，可致咳逆不已、痰粘色黄、咳吐不利等症。如《血证论•咳血》曰: "盖肺金火甚，则煎熬水液为痰，水液伤，则肺叶不能腴润下垂，其在下之肝肾，气又熏之，肺叶焦举，不胜制节，故气逆为咳，气愈逆，所以久咳不止也。" 治宜滋阴清热，润肺止咳。方选《医学心悟》月华丸（沙参、麦冬、天冬、生地、熟地、阿胶、桑叶、菊花、川贝母、百部、山药、茯苓、三七、獭肝）; 若肺阴亏虚，肺火日盛，热迫血行，损伤肺络，可致咳逆胸痛、痰中带血，或咯出鲜红色血液。诚如《景岳全书•杂证谟•血证》说: "凡病血者，虽有五脏之辨，然无不由于水亏，水亏则火盛，火盛则刑金，金病则肺燥，肺燥则络伤易嗽血，液涸而成痰。" 《血证论•咳血》也说: "肺为娇脏，无论外感内伤，但一伤其津液，则阴虚火动，肺中被刑，金失清肃下降之令，其气上逆，嗽痰咳血。" 肺虚火炎，虚火伤络，热迫血行，随咳而出，便为咳血。治宜滋阴清热，凉血止血。方选《证治要诀》白芨枇杷膏（生地黄、阿胶、白芨、藕节、枇杷叶）加白茅根、侧柏叶、仙鹤草、小蓟、血余炭；此外，肺阴不足，虚火内生可引起全身性虚热症，表现为全身低热、五心烦热、午后潮热、颧红盗汗等热象。治宜滋阴清热。方选《证治准绳》清骨散（银柴胡、胡黄连、青蒿、地骨皮、秦艽、鳖甲）加生地黄。

Literature Review of Yīn Vacuity Flaming Fire

📖 *Míng Yī Zá Zhù* ("Miscellaneous Works by Famous Physicians"), "Taxation Consumption"

> "Excessive sexual desire damages essence and blood and will invariably engender the disease of yīn vacuity stirring fire. The symptoms of night sweating during sleep, postmeridial heat effusion, hacking cough, fatigue and lack of strength, low intake of food and drink, in severe cases phlegm-drool containing blood, expectoration and ejection of blood, possibly coughing of blood, blood ejection, or nosebleed; generalized heat effusion, a sunken rapid pulse, and emaciation of the flesh, all these are a condition called taxation consumption."

This quotation describes the important pathomechanism by which essence-blood depletion, yīn vacuity stirring fire, and vacuity heat harassing internally and forcing blood to move frenetically leads to cough, blood ejection, and tidal heat and night sweating.

📖 *Zhèng Zhì Huì Bǔ* ("Combined Supplements to Patterns and Treatment"), "Cough"

> "Yīn vacuity cough means vexing heat in the five hearts and qì ascending together with fire, which worsens in the afternoon and at night."

This quotation indicates the pathomechanism by which yīn vacuity and failure to restrain yáng makes vacuity fire arise internally. When this rises and harasses the lung, it leads to qì counterflow and cough; when it harasses the entire body, it leads to vexing heat in thc fivc hearts. At the same time, this source stresses that these symptoms occur mostly in the afternoon or at night.

📖 *Zhèng Yīn Mài Zhì* ("Pathoconditions: Causes, Pulses, and Treatments"), "Cough"

> "The signs of blood vacuity cough are night sweating and spontaneous sweating, tidal heat and steaming bone, increased cough in the afternoon, black and emaciated body, and vexing heat in the five heart."

Blood vacuity means yīn vacuity, and when yīn is vacuous, yáng becomes hyperactive. When vacuity fire harasses the upper body, lung qì ascends counterflow, resulting in cough. When it harasses the entire body, the result is tidal heat, night sweating, steaming bone, and vexing heat in the five hearts.

📖 *Lǐ Xū Yuán Jiàn* ("The Original Mirror of Rectifying Vacuity"), "Yīn Vacuity Conditions are Associated with the Lung"

> "There are conditions that gradually proceed from steaming bone to taxation cough. There are conditions that gradually proceed from taxation cough to blood ejection. There are conditions that unexpectedly manifest with steaming bone and desiccation, and subsequent death, without first forming taxation cough. There are conditions that begin with taxation cough and are accompanied by blood ejection. Lastly, there are conditions that begin with blood ejection and are accompanied by taxation cough… All of these can be treated completely through the lung. The reason for this is that yīn vacuity taxation damage, while also called 'five taxations and seven damages,' can be summed up as the lung is the supreme principle."

This quotation discusses the effects of yīn vacuity internal heat: Harassing the lung, it can cause taxation cough; harassing the entire body, it can cause steaming bone heat effusion; forcing blood to move, it can cause blood ejection.

文献评述

《明医杂著•劳瘵》曰: "色欲过度，损伤精血，必生阴虚火动之病。睡中盗汗，午后发热，哈哈咳嗽，倦怠无力，饮食少进，甚则痰涎带血，咯吐出血，或咳血、吐血、衄血，身热，脉沉数，肌肉消瘦，此名劳瘵。" 论述了精血亏损，阴虚火动，虚热内扰，迫血妄行，引起咳嗽、吐血、潮热盗汗的重要病机。

《证治汇补•咳嗽》曰: "阴虚咳嗽者，五心烦热，气从火升，午后夜甚，" 指出阴虚，阴不制阳，虚火内生，上扰于肺，引起气逆咳嗽; 内扰全身，引起五心烦热的病机。并指出此类现象，多发于午后或夜间。

《症因脉治•咳嗽》曰: "血虚咳嗽之症，盗汗自汗，潮热骨蒸，下午嗽多，形体黑瘦，五心烦热" 血虚应为阴虚，阴虚阳亢，虚火上扰，肺气上逆而咳; 虚热扰动全身，则潮热盗汗骨蒸，五心烦热。

《理虚元鉴•阴虚之证统于肺》曰: "有从骨蒸而渐至劳嗽者，有从劳嗽而渐至吐血者，有竟以骨蒸枯竭而死，不待成劳嗽者，有竟从劳嗽起，而兼吐血者，有竟从吐血起，而兼劳嗽者。…凡此种种，悉宰于肺治。所以然者，阴虚劳伤，虽有五劳、七伤之异名，而要之以肺为极则。”论述了阴虚内热，上扰于肺，可致劳嗽；内扰全身，可致骨蒸发热；热迫血行，可致吐血。

Summary of Yīn Vacuity Flaming Fire
1. Vacuity Fire Harassing the Upper Body Incessant cough and counterflow, sticky yellow phlegm, inhibited coughing and spitting. 2. Heat Distressing the Movement of Blood Cough and counterflow with chest pain, phlegm containing bright red blood. 3. Generalized Vacuity Heat Generalized low-grade fever, vexing heat in the five hearts, postmeridian tidal heat, reddening of the cheeks and night sweating.

阴虚火炎
虚火上扰——咳逆不已、痰粘色黄、咳吐不利。 热迫血行——咳逆胸痛、痰中带血，血色鲜红。 全身虚热——全身低热、五心烦热、午后潮热、颧红盗汗。

When the pathomechanism of lung yīn vacuity progresses to a more advanced state, it can lead to such pathomechanical changes as lung-stomach yīn vacuity and lung-kidney yīn vacuity.

Lung-Stomach Yīn Vacuity

The lung is metal and the spleen is earth. When lung yīn vacuity progresses further, the child can steal the mother's qì, and damage can thus affect stomach yīn. When stomach yīn is vacuous, earth fails to engender metal, which can also lead to lung yīn vacuity. Interacting as mutual cause and effect, this can form the pathomechanism of lung-stomach yīn vacuity. It manifests in the simultaneous appearance of dry cough with scant phlegm and ungratifying expectoration of phlegm, together with hunger with no desire to eat, discomfort in the stomach duct, and dry retching and hiccup. This condition is treated by enriching and nourishing lung and stomach yīn. The recommended formula is *shā shēn mài dōng tāng* (Adenophora/glehnia and Ophiopogon Decoction from the *Wēn Bìng Tiáo Bian* ("Systematized Identification of Warm Diseases").

Shā Shēn Mài Dōng Tāng 沙参麦冬汤 (Adenophora/glehnia and Ophiopogon Decoction)
shā shēn 沙参 (Adenophorae seu Glehniae Radix, adenophora/glehnia) *mài mén dōng* 麦门冬 (Ophiopogonis Radix, ophiopogon) *yù zhú* 玉竹 (Polygonati Odorati Rhizoma, Solomon's seal) *tiān huā fěn* 天花粉 (Trichosanthis Radix, trichosanthes root) *bái biǎn dòu* 白扁豆 (Lablab Semen Album, lablab) *sāng yè* 桑叶 (Mori Folium, mulberry leaf) *gān cǎo* 甘草 (Glycyrrhizae Radix, licorice)

Lung-Kidney Yīn Vacuity

The lung is metal and the kidney is water. When lung yīn is insufficient, the disease of the mother can affect the child. If metal fails to engender water, damage can thus affect kidney yīn, forming the pathomechanism of lung-kidney yīn vacuity. It manifests in the symptoms of cough with scant phlegm, exhalation more than inhalation, limp aching lumbus and knees, and seminal emission and insomnia. When lung yīn is insufficient and liquid fails to transform qì, this can lead to lung qì debilitation and form the pathomechanism of dual vacuity of lung qì and lung yīn. It manifests in panting and cough, scant thick and sticky phlegm, ungratifying coughing of phlegm with low sound, fatigued spirit and lack of strength, tidal heat, and night sweating. Lung-kidney yīn vacuity is treated by enriching and supplementing lung and kidney yīn. The recommended formula is *mài wèi dì huáng tāng* (Ophiopogonis, Schisandra, Rehmanniae Decoction) from the *Yī Zōng Jīn Jiàn* ("The Golden Mirror of Medicine").

Mài Wèi Dì Huáng Tāng 麦味地黄汤 (Ophiopogonis, Schisandra, and Rehmanniae Decoction)
shú dì huáng 熟地黄 (Rehmanniae Radix Praeparata, cooked rehmannia) *shān zhū yú* 山茱萸 (Corni Fructus, cornus) *shān yào* 山药 (Dioscoreae Rhizoma, dioscorea) *zé xiè* 泽泻 (Alismatis Rhizoma, alisma) *fú líng* 茯苓 (Poria, poria) *mǔ dān pí* 牡丹皮 (Moutan Cortex, moutan) *mài mén dōng* 麦门冬 (Ophiopogonis Radix, ophiopogon) *wǔ wèi zǐ* 五味子 (Schisandrae Fructus, schisandra)

肺阴虚的病机进一步发展，可引起肺胃阴虚，肺肾阴虚等病机变化。

肺胃阴虚: 肺金胃土，肺阴虚进一步演化，子盗母气，可伤及胃阴；胃阴虚，土不生金，亦可引起肺阴虚，两者互为因果，形成肺胃阴虚的病机。出现干咳痰少，咯痰不爽与饥不欲食，胃脘不舒、干呕呃逆等症同见。治宜滋养肺胃之阴。方选《温病条辨》沙参麦冬汤。

肺肾阴虚: 肺金肾水，肺阴不足，母病及子，金不生水，可伤及肾阴，形成肺肾阴虚的病机。表现为咳嗽痰少、呼多吸少、腰膝酸软、遗精失眠等症。肺阴不足，津不化气，可致肺气虚衰，形成肺的气阴两虚的病机, 则可见咳嗽气喘、痰少粘稠、咳痰声低不爽、神疲乏力、潮热盗汗等症。治宜滋补肺肾之阴。方选《医宗金鉴》麦味地黄汤（熟地、山茱萸、山药、泽泻、茯苓、丹皮、麦冬、五味子）。

Chapter Seven

Lung Blood Vacuity

Historically, the pathomechanism of lung blood vacuity was mentioned only rarely, with the result that most people were not aware of the existence of lung blood vacuity patterns. Numerous scholars pointed out that since the lung assembles the hundred vessels and is always filled with an abundance of blood, it could therefore not develop the pathomechanism of lung blood vacuity. If we follow this line of reasoning, since the heart governs the blood and vessels, and the liver stores blood, these two viscera are also abundantly supplied with blood and should not develop the pathomechanisms of heart blood vacuity or liver blood vacuity either.

Obviously, these ideas do not rest on sufficient theoretical evidence. Every viscus and bowel in the human body can be affected by pathomechanical changes in the aspects of qì, blood, yīn, and yáng. During the time that the lung is involved in a substantial number of physiological functions, it is impossible that lung blood would not suffer damage. In other words, in clinical practice this should objectively result in the pathomechanical changes of lung blood vacuity. The reason why it has been ignored for such a long time is that the pathomechanical changes of lung blood vacuity are not very obvious and furthermore tend to occur simultaneously with the pathomechanisms of lung qì vacuity and lung yīn vacuity. Thus they are easily concealed by their pathomechanisms and clinical manifestations. Because the differentiation and diagnosis of lung blood vacuity are difficult, it has not easily gained wide-spread acceptance.

Before the Táng period, discussions that involved lung blood vacuity were extremely rare. From the Sòng period on, however, the pathomechanical changes of lung vacuity began to be discussed from the angle of qì and blood vacuity. For example, Wáng Huái-Yǐn stated in the chapter, "Cough" in the *Tài Píng Shèng Huì Fāng* ("The Great Peace Sagacious Benevolence Formulary"):

> "Enduring cough is caused by extreme lung vacuity. If lung qì is vacuous, it is struck by wind-cold. Over years and months, this results in cough.

> This is always related to disharmony between yīn and yáng, to vacuity of qì and blood, and to wind-cold qì striking the channels and network vessels and accumulating inside the body. As right and evil struggle with each other, they congest and astringe the pathways of qì, which results in cough that does not improve for a long period of time."

In this quotation, vacuity of qì and blood does not only indicate lung qì vacuity, but also includes lung blood vacuity.

In "Treatise on Cough Formulas" in the *Rén Zhāi Zhí Zhǐ Fù Yí Fāng Lùn* ("Supplement to 'Rén-Zhāi Clear Guidance Formulary"), Yáng Shì-Yíng stated:

> "Vacuity taxation causes scantness of blood, internal consumption of fluids, and upflaming of heart fire. Consequently, dryness-heat overwhelms the lung, causing expectoration and spitting of pus and blood, and tidal ascent of qì and drool. The cough will be continuous and incessant. Should blood fail to luxuriate the flesh, evil in the skin and body hair is able to enter the lung, with particular speed if it is contracted from the back. In that case, you must use *rén shēn xiōng guī tāng* (Ginseng, Chuan Xiong, and Angelica Decoction)."

This quotation not only mentions "vacuity taxation causing scantness of blood" directly as a cause of incessant cough, but it also illustrates rather clearly the pathomechanism by which blood vacuity and inability to nourish the skin, and evil qì exploiting vacuity and entering the lung form lung blood vacuity, which results in cough.

In the chapter, "Cough" in the Míng dynasty text *Yī Xué Zhèng Zhuàn* ("The Orthodox Tradition of Medicine"), Yú Tuán stated: "Cough with a hoarse sound means that blood is vacuous and has contracted heat." He further stated: "Cough with a stringlike rough pulse means scant blood." When commenting on *xìng sū sǎn* (Apricot Kernel and Perilla Powder), he clearly pointed out the symptoms, pulse manifestation, and treatment method for cough caused by lung blood vacuity:

> "For blood vacuity with phlegm, use this formula in combination with *sì wù tāng* (Four Agents Decoction) and with the addition of *wǔ wèi zǐ* (Schisandrae Fructus), *mài mén dōng* (Ophiopogonis Radix), and *guā lōu rén* (Trichosanthis Semen)."

In the chapter, "Blood Vacuity Cough" in the *Zhèng Yīn Mài Zhì* ("Pathoconditions: Causes, Pulses, and Treatments"), Qín Chāng-Yù further pointed out:

> "[Blood vacuity cough is caused by] yīn blood depletion and yīn vacuity, which results in internal heat. Boiling true yīn, yīn fire becomes daily more exuberant, restrains lung metal, and thereby causes the symptom of cough. … [When the pulse manifests as] a fine rapid pulse on the left inch position, lung yīn has suffered detriment and center qì is vacuous, such that qì fails to engender blood."

The Qīng Dynasty author Píng Zhào-Zhāng analyzed vacuity cough in the chapter, “Combined Investigation of Prescriptions, Pulses, and Symptoms of Cough” in the *Féng Shì Jǐn Náng Mì Lù* (“Feng’s Secret Record of the Brocade Pouch”). Among two types, he characterized one as “night cough with increased thirst, phlegm that is not easily expectorated, and heat effusion. This is blood vacuity.” Here, he further clarified the special characteristic that cough caused by lung blood vacuity occurs most prominently at night and manifests as dry cough with scant phlegm that is not easily expectorated, with simultaneous heat effusion and thirst.

In the chapter, “Cough” in the *Yī Zōng Yǐ Rèn Biān* (“Transmission of Medical Orthodoxy”), the Qīng period author Gāo Gǔ-Fēng stated: “Afternoon cough is related to yīn blood vacuity. Treat it with *sì wù tāng* (Four Agents Decoction), with the addition of *jiǔ bàn chǎo huáng bái* (wine-fried Cortex Phellodendri) and *zhī mǔ* (Anemarrhenae Rhizoma).” He pointed out that the representative formula for treating lung blood vacuity is *sì wù tāng* (Four Agents Decoction).

The sources cited above show that early physicians mostly discussed lung blood vacuity in conjunction with lung yīn vacuity or lung qì vacuity, referring to it summarily as qì-blood or yīn-blood, and very rarely discussed lung blood vacuity in isolation. Therefore, most people were extremely unfamiliar with this pathomechanism. It was only in the 1990s that representative academic monographs in textbooks on basic theory and visceral manifestation included formal descriptions of lung blood vacuity.

Factors that cause lung blood vacuity include enduring or severe illness damaging yīn blood; spleen-stomach vacuity, preventing engenderment of new blood; bleeding patterns like blood ejection or nosebleed causing lung blood insufficiency; and taxation damage or consumption worms eroding the lung and causing lung blood depletion. The most important pathomechanism of lung blood vacuity is blood vacuity with failure to moisten.

Lung blood vacuity can lead to serious clinical symptoms like cough, phlegm that is not easily expectorated, expectoration of blood or of phlegm containing blood, shortage of qì and hasty panting that is lighter during the day and more severe at night, pale facial complexion, mouth, lips, and nails, absence of or reduced sweating, dizzy head and flowery vision, pale white tongue, and a fine pulse.

The lung is the delicate viscus. When lung blood is insufficient and fails to moisten, the lung loses its ability to carry out diffusion and depurative downbearing, and lung qì ascends counterflow, causing panting and cough. When lung blood is insufficient and blood fails to nourish liquid, it causes dry cough with scant phlegm that is not easily expectorated, dry mouth and throat, and a hoarse voice. When lung blood is vacuous and therefore unable to transform qì, lung qì becomes insufficient and ancestral qì is debilitated, resulting in cough and panting with shortness of breath, heart palpitations, and fearful throbbing.

This condition is treated by nourishing blood and moistening dryness. The recommended formula is *sì wù tāng* (Four Agents Decoction) in combination with a variation of *shēng mài sǎn* (Pulse-Engendering Powder).

Sì Wù Tāng 四物汤 (Four Agents Decoction)
dāng guī 当归 (Angelicae Sinensis Radix, Chinese angelica) *shú dì huáng* 熟地黄 (Rehmanniae Radix Praeparata, cooked rehmannia) *sháo yào* 芍药 (Paeoniae Radix, peony) *chuān xiōng* 川芎 (Chuanxiong Rhizoma, chuanxiong)

Shēng Mài Sǎn 生脉散 (Pulse-Engendering Powder)
rén shēn 人参 (Ginseng Radix, ginseng) *mài mén dōng* 麦门冬 (Ophiopogonis Radix, ophiopogon) *wǔ wèi zǐ* 五味子 (Schisandrae Fructus, schisandra)

If lung blood insufficiency prevents yīn from restraining yáng, vacuity heat harasses internally, resulting in cough that is lighter during the day and more severe at night. If enduring cough damages the network vessels or consumption worms erode the lung, the result is expectoration of blood or of phlegm containing blood. When lung blood is vacuous and therefore unable to ascend and nourish the head and face, the result is dizzy head and flowery vision, pale white facial complexion, pale mouth and lips and nails, and a pale tender-soft white tongue. Inability to nourish the blood in the vessels results in a fine pulse. This condition is treated by nourishing blood and moistening the lung, and by quieting the network vessels and stanching bleeding. The recommended formula is *rén shēn xiōng guī tāng* (Ginseng, Chuan Xiong, Angelicae Decoction) from the *Zhí Zhǐ Fāng* ("Direct Guide to Formulas").

Rén Shēn Xiōng Guī Tāng 人参芎归汤 (Ginseng, Chuan Xiong, and Angelicae Decoction)
dāng guī 当归 (Angelicae Sinensis Radix, Chinese angelica) *chuān xiōng* 川芎 (Chuanxiong Rhizoma, chuanxiong) *bái sháo* 白芍 (Paeoniae Radix, Alba, white peony) *rén shēn* 人参 (Ginseng Radix, ginseng)

bàn xià 半夏 (Pinelliae Rhizoma, pinellia)
jú pí 橘皮 (Citri Fructus Pericarpium)
chì fú líng 赤茯苓 (Poria Rubra, red poria)
ē jiāo 阿胶 (Asini Corii Colla, ass hide glue)
xì xīn 细辛 (Asari Radix, asarum)
wǔ wèi zǐ 五味子 (Schisandrae Fructus, schisandra)
gān cǎo 甘草 (Glycyrrhizae Radix, licorice)

肺血虚

肺血虚的病机历来提及甚少，以致多数人认为不存在肺血虚证。不少学者提出: 肺朝百脉，肺中血液十分丰富，不可能发生肺血虚的病机变化。如此推理，心主血脉，肝藏血，心肝二脏血液充足，均不应有心血虚、肝血虚的病机。显然上述说法没有充足的理论依据。人体每一脏腑都应有气血阴阳的病机变化，肺脏在从事大量生理功能活动的同时，不可能不发生肺血的损伤。也就是说，在临床实践中，客观上应当引起肺血虚的病机变化。之所以长期以来未引起人们的重视，是因为肺血虚的病机变化不太显著，又常与肺气虚、肺阴虚的病机同时发生，容易被肺气虚、肺阴虚的病机及临床表现所掩盖，鉴别诊断比较困难，故不容易获得大家的公认。

唐代以前极少涉及肺血虚的论述，宋代开始，从气血虚弱的角度阐述肺虚的病机变化。如王怀隐《太平圣惠方•咳嗽》云: “夫久咳嗽者，由肺虚极故也。肺气既虚，为风寒所搏，连滞岁月而咳嗽也。此皆阴阳不调，气血虚弱，风冷之气搏于经络，留积于内，邪正相并，气道壅涩，则咳嗽而经久不差也。”其中气血虚弱，不仅指肺气虚，也包括了肺血虚。杨士瀛《仁斋直指附遗方论•咳嗽方论》云“虚劳血少，津液内耗，心火上炎，遂使燥热乘肺，咯唾脓血，上气涎潮，其咳嗽连续而不已。惟夫血不荣肌，故邪在皮毛，皆能入肺，而自背得之尤速，则人参芎归所不可无。”其中不仅直接提出“虚劳血少”是引起咳嗽不已的病因，还较为清楚地阐明血虚不能营养肌肤，邪气乘虚入肺，是肺血虚导致咳嗽的病机。明代虞抟《医学正传•咳嗽》云: “咳嗽声嘶者，乃血虚受热。”又云: “脉弦涩而咳，为少血。”并在杏苏饮下云: “血虚有痰者，本方合四物汤加五味子、麦门冬、瓜蒌仁之类。”明确指出了肺血虚所致咳嗽的症状、脉象和治法。秦昌遇《症因脉治•血虚咳嗽》中进一步指出血虚咳嗽的病因为“形役阳亢，阴血亏损，血虚则内热，煎熬真阴，阴火日旺，肺金被克，而咳嗽之症作矣”。其脉象“左寸细数，肺阴有损，中气虚弱，气不生血。”清代冯兆张《冯氏锦囊秘录•方脉咳嗽合参》中分析虚嗽有二，其中“夜嗽多口渴，痰不易出，发热为血虚。”，更点明肺血虚所致咳嗽的时间特征多在夜间，症状为干咳痰少，不易咯出，兼发热、口渴等症。清代高鼓峰《医宗已任编•咳嗽》云：“午后咳嗽属阴血虚，四物汤加酒拌炒黄柏、知母。”提出治疗肺血虚的代表方剂为四物汤。从上可以看出，古代医家大多把肺血虚与肺阴虚或肺气虚相提并论，统称气血或阴血，很少单独提出肺血虚的论述，故大家对肺血虚的病机感到十分陌生。直到 90 年代末期，在《中医藏象学》及《中医药学高级丛书•中医基础理论》等代表性学术专著中才相继有肺血虚的正式论述。引起肺血虚的病因包括久病，重病耗伤阴血；脾胃虚弱，不能化生新血；吐血、衄血各种失血病证，导致肺血不足；劳伤或痨虫蚀肺，致使肺血亏损。肺血虚的病机主要为血少失濡。

肺血虚可引起咳嗽，痰不易出，咯血，或痰中带血，少气喘促，日轻夜重，面色、口唇、爪甲色淡；无汗或少汗，头晕眼花，舌淡白，脉细等主要临床表现。

肺为娇脏，肺血不足，失于濡养，肺失宣发肃降，肺气上逆，则咳嗽气喘；肺血不足，血不养津，故干咳少痰，不易咯出，口干咽燥，声音嘶哑。肺血虚少，不能化气，肺气不足，宗气衰少则咳喘气短，心悸，怔忡。治宜养血润燥，方选四物汤合生脉散加减。若肺血不足，阴不制阳，虚热内扰，则咳嗽，日轻夜重；久咳伤络，或痨虫蚀肺，则咯血或痰中带血；肺血虚，不能上养于头面，则头晕眼花，面色淡白，口唇、爪甲色淡，舌质嫩淡白；不能充养血脉，则脉细。法当养血润肺，宁络止血。方用《直指方》人参芎归汤（当归、川芎、白芍、人参、半夏、橘皮、赤茯苓、阿胶、细辛、北五味、甘草）。

Literature Review of Lung Blood Vacuity

📖 *Rén Zhāi Zhí Zhǐ Fù Yí Fāng Lùn* (“Supplement to ‘Rén Zhāi Clear Guidance Formulary”), “Treatise on Cough Formulas”

> “*Rén shēn xiōng guī tāng* (Ginseng, Chuan Xiong, and Angelica Decoction): treats vacuity taxation and scantness of blood, internal consumption of fluids, spontaneous flaming of heart fire, dryness-heat overwhelming the lung, cough with ejection of blood, as well as blood failing to luxuriate the flesh and at the slightest physical exertion, cold [contracted through] the body hair and cough.”

This quotation points out that lung blood vacuity prevents blood from nourishing the skin, flesh, and body hair. This makes external defense insecure and allows external evils to easily invade the lung, resulting in cough. At the same time, it also describes how scanty blood and depleted fluids allow vacuity fire to harass the inner body, which can lead to cough and expectoration of blood.

🕮 *Yī Xué Zhèng Zhuàn* ("The Orthodox Tradition of Medicine"), "Cough"

"For cough with yīn vacuity stirring fire, use *sì wù tāng* (Four Agents Decoction) in combination with *èr chén tāng* (Two Matured Ingredients Decoction), to smooth and precipitate it." "Yīn vacuity cough with spitting red is treated with *sì wù tāng* (Four Agents Decoction) with the addition of *zhī mǔ* (Anemarrhenae Rhizoma), *huáng bǎi* (Phellodendri Cortex), *wǔ wèi zǐ* (Schisandrae Fructus), *rén shēn* (Ginseng Radix), *mài mén dōng* (Ophiopogonis Radix), *sāng bái pí* (Mori Cortex), and *dì gǔ pí* (Lycii Cortex)."

If yīn vacuity in these two instances only referred to cough and expectoration of blood from yīn liquid depletion, the author would have recommended treating them with yīn-nourishing, heat-clearing, and blood-stanching formulas like *shā shēn mài dōng tāng* (Adenophora/glehnia and Ophiopogon Decoction) or *bǎi hé gù jīn tāng* (Lily Bulb Metal-Securing Decoction). However, the fact that the author uses variations of *sì wù tāng* (Four Agents Decoction) shows that these conditions also include the pathomechanism of lung blood vacuity.

🕮 *Míng Yī Zá Zhù* ("Miscellaneous Works by Famous Physicians"), "Cough"

"Productive cough in the afternoon is related to yīn vacuity, which means taxation cough. It is treated by supplementing yīn and downbearing fire. Add *chuān xiōng* (Chuanxiong Rhizoma), *dāng guī* (Angelicae Sinensis Radix), *sháo yào* (Paeoniae Radix), *shú dì huáng* (Rehmanniae Radix Praeparata), *huáng bǎi* (Phellodendri Cortex), *zhī mǔ* (Anemarrhenae Rhizoma), *zhú lì* (Bambusae Succus), *tiān dōng* (Asparagi Radix), *guā lóu zǐ* (Trichosanthis Semen), and *bèi mǔ* (Fritillariae Bulbus). This formula specifically supplements yīn-blood."

This formula uses a variation of *sì wù tāng* (Four Agents Decoction) to treat afternoon cough. By emphasizing that it "specifically supplements yīn-blood," it explains that afternoon cough is caused by an insufficiency of yīn-blood. Blood is yīn, and the afternoon is related to yīn. Therefore cough that is caused by yīn-blood depletion tends to occur in the afternoon.

🕮 *Yī Mén Fǎ Lǜ* ("Axioms of Medicine"), "Treatise on Cough"

"Either construction blood is debilitated and therefore unable to nourish the sinews, or essence and marrow are consumed and therefore unable to fill the bones. Either of these cause lung-metal to dry out more every day. Fire enters without any resistance, causing cough without respite. At this time, urgently engender liquid, supplement blood, and supplement essence and water, and you can still treat it. But if you fail to do this and do not treat it, in a blink of an eye the jar will be dry and the cup empty,

> causing brittle hair and sickly complexion, tense sinews and dry nails, tautness in the chest and back, upward pulling pain in both rib-sides, lung qì huffing and depression, all sorts of wilting, panting, and retching, congested throat with bloody discharge, and all sorts of critical signs that are interrelated."

Yīn and blood are of the same source. Debilitation of construction-blood and essence and marrow both mean scant blood failing to moisten. When lung blood is insufficient, lung-metal is dry and depuration breaks down, causing incessant cough. Therefore treatment needs to be swift to engender essence and supplement blood. Otherwise the condition is likely to lead to critical symptoms like cough, counterflow, panting, and wilting. Here Dr. Yù expounds to great depth the complex pathomechanical changes resulting from lung blood vacuity.

🕮 *Féng Shì Jǐn Náng Mì Lù* ("Feng's Secret Record of the Brocade Pouch"), "Combined Investigation of Prescriptions, Pulses, and Symptoms in Cough."

> "Cough with phlegm and qì ascent is mostly caused by an insufficiency of yīn blood and by trouble from vacuity fire and vacuity qì floating upward. Wanting to dissipate the phlegm, you will exhaust blood. Wanting to move qì, you will further discharge the origin…
>
> After phlegm is opened [as a result of treatment with phlegm-expelling medicinals, lung qì only gets] blocked again. If you use blood-engendering medicinals, [they will make lung qì] descend from Heaven, and over days in the course of time cause blood to be engendered. When blood is engendered, qì returns to the blood chamber, just like a prodigal son returning home, able to restore the family business."

This quotation points out that yīn blood insufficiency in the lung and vacuity fire harassing the upper body is an important pathomechanism that causes cough and qì counterflow. At the same time, the fact that it discusses supplementing lung blood to cause lung qì to recover and to obtain improvement for signs such as cough and qì counterflow serves as counterevidence for the objective existence of the pathomechanism of lung blood vacuity.

文献评述

《仁斋直指附遗方论•咳嗽方论》曰: "人参芎归汤: 治虚劳血少，津液内耗，心火自炎，燥热乘肺，咳嗽咯血，及血不荣肌，动辄毛寒咳嗽。" 指出肺血虚，血不营养肌肤、皮毛，卫外不固，外邪容易犯肺而引起咳嗽；同时又论述血少津亏，虚火内扰，可致咳嗽咯血。

《医学正传•咳嗽》曰: "阴虚火动而咳嗽，四物合二陈，顺而下之。" "阴虚喘嗽而吐红者，四物加知母、黄柏、五味子、人参、麦门冬、桑白皮、地骨皮。”两处阴虚，若单指阴津亏损所致咳嗽咯血，则当用沙参麦冬、百合固金汤等养阴清热止血的方剂治疗。此处选四物汤加减，说明应包含肺血虚的病机在内。

《明医杂著•咳嗽》曰:“若午后嗽者，属阴虚，即劳嗽也，宜补阴降火，加川芎、当归、芍药、熟地、黄柏、知母、竹沥、天门冬、瓜蒌仁、贝母，此专补阴血也。”此方用四物汤加减，治疗午后咳嗽，并指出“专补阴血”，说明午后咳嗽，为阴血不足所致。血为阴，午后属阴，故以阴血亏损所致咳嗽在午后容易发生。

《医门法律•咳嗽论》曰:“或营血衰少，不养于筋;或精髓耗竭，不充于骨，乃致肺金日久干燥，火入莫御，咳无止息。此时亟生其津，亟补其血，亟补其精水，犹可为也。失此不治，转盼瓮干杯罄，毛瘁色弊，筋急爪枯，咳引胸背，吊胁疼痛，肺气膹郁，诸痿喘呕，嗌塞血泄，种种危象，相因而见。”精血同源，营血、精髓衰少，均为血少失濡。肺血不足，肺金干燥，清肃失职，故咳无休止，故治疗应迅速生精补血，否则容易引起咳逆喘痿等多种危重证候。喻氏极其深刻地论述肺血虚可引起的复杂病机变化。

《冯氏锦囊秘录•方脉咳嗽合参》曰:“夫咳嗽生痰上气，多因阴血不足，虚火虚气上浮而为患也。欲消其痰，转耗其血;欲行其气，更泄其元。…迨至痰之开而复闭，而所用生血之药，早已从天而降，日续一日，久久而血生，血生而气返血室，如浪子归家，复能振作立业。”指出肺的阴血不足，虚火上扰，是引起咳嗽气逆的重要病机。并通过补肺血，使肺气恢复，咳嗽气逆等症可得以好转，从而反证肺血虚病机的客观存在。

Summary of Blood Failing to Nourish

1. Impairing Diffusion and Depuration

   Cough and panting, dry cough with scant phlegm that is not easily expectorated, dry mouth and hoarse voice.

2. Inability to Transform Qì

   Cough with panting and shortness of breath, heart palpitations, fearful throbbing.

3. Blood Vacuity Transforming into Heat

   Cough that is lighter during the day and more severe at night.

4. Enduring Cough Damaging the Network Vessels

   Expectoration of blood or of phlegm containing blood.

5. Head and Face Deprived of Nourishment

   Dizzy head and flowery vision, pale white facial complexion, pale mouth, lips, and nails, tender-soft pale white tongue.

血失滋养
失于宣肃——咳嗽气喘，干咳少痰，不易咯出，口干声嘶。
不能化气——咳喘气短，心悸，怔忡。
血虚化热——咳嗽，日轻夜重。
久咳伤络——咯血或痰中带血。
头面失养——头晕眼花，面色淡白，口唇、爪甲色淡，舌嫩淡白。

It is relatively rare that the pathomechanism of lung blood vacuity appears in isolation, and it is much more frequently observed together with lung qì vacuity or lung yīn vacuity. Therefore, when you are engaged in the process of identifying patterns of lung disease in the clinic, you will certainly have to consider the pathomechanism of lung blood vacuity to avoid a number of blunders or incomplete diagnosis in clinic when identifying patterns as the basis for determining treatment.

肺血虚病机单独出现的时间较少，但与肺气虚、肺阴虚同时并见的机会很多。故临床从事肺病辨证的时候，一定要考虑肺血虚的病机，否则在临床辨证论治容易引起许多错误或漏诊。

Bibliography of Chinese Sources

Journals and Periodicals

1. 郭一清等.肺气虚与肺扫描、肺功能的关系, 上海中医药杂志, 1984, (9): 47
2. 林求诚.慢阻肺中医辨证的诊断学意义, 北京中医学院学报, 1984, (5): 21
3. 王会仍等.从心肺功能变化看肺气与心血的关系, 浙江中医杂, 1987, 22(1): 25
4. 苏梅者等.慢性咳喘病中医辨证与肺功能关系的研究, 中医杂志, 1990, 31(3): 49
5. 周庆伟等.血神口服液对“慢阻肺”肺气虚证患者微量元素及肺功能变化的临床研究, 河南中医, 1 996, 16（2）: 18.
6. 徐锡鸿等.肺气虚与气道反应性关系探讨, 辽宁中医杂志, 1996, 23（2）, 66.
7. 李力等.I 期煤工尘肺肺气虚患者肺功能测定结果分析, 北京中医药大学学报, 1 996, 19（6）: 48
8. 柴秀娟等.哮喘病肺气虚与气道反应性关系初探, 浙江中医杂志, 1997, （5）: 219.
9. 赵勤萍等.补肺止嗽胶囊治疗慢性支气管炎肺气虚证 53 例疗效观察, 山西中医, 1998, l4（3）: 9.
10. 徐锡鸣等.哮喘肺气虚患者情志因素与气道反应性关系的探讨.福建中医药, 1999, 30（4）: 1 1
11. 陈乐宏, 肾资血、肺行血初探, 山东中医学院学报, 1983(1): 25
12. 江丹.近年来气虚证客观诊断指标的研究进展, 北京中医学院学报, 1984, (2): 45
13. 宋崇顺.气虚证血液流变学的临床观察和实验研究, 中医杂志, 1981; 22（10）: 39
14. 广西中医学院中医理论研究室. 肺气虚的实质研究, 广西中医药, 1981, (4): 33

15. 何权瀛.肺气虚的实质的研究, 中西医结合杂志, 1985, 5(5): 618
16. 宋崇顺等.气虚证血液流变学的临床观察和实验研究, 中医杂志 , 1981, (10): 39
17. 金维岳等.慢性支气管炎、肺源性心脏病患者血液流变学检查与中西医结合临床分型的关系, 江西医药, 1982, (3): 49
18. 杨牧祥等.实验性 SD 大鼠'肺气虚证'血液流变学改变和免疫功能状态研究, 河北中医, 1996, (5): 42
19. 林求诚."慢阻肺"中医辨证的诊断学意义, 北京中医学院学报, 1984; （5）: 21
20. 王素英等.肺心病辨证分型应用血气、心肺功能、超声心动图的意义, 内蒙古中医药, 1986, (3): 26
21. 靖旭荔等.肺心病中西医结合辨证分型 202 例次血气、酸碱和电解质变化规律探讨, 中西医结合杂志, 1985, (8): 466
22. 李莹.40 例肺气虚患者血液流变学、甲皱微循环测定, 辽宁中医杂志, 1992; 19（6）: 6
23. 王会仍等.肺气虚与慢性阻塞性肺病关系及其本质的研究, .中国医药学报, 1992, 7（4）: 62.
24. 王元勋等.肺气虚证的实验研究III—血液流变学及血浆 TXB2、6—keto—PGF1α 水平的临床研究, 甘肃中医学院学报, 1994, 11（1）: 52
25. 杨牧祥等.补气方、活血方、补气活血方对肺气虚证患者血液流变学的影响, 中国中医基础医学杂志, 1997, 3（6）: 42
26. 刘畅.全国首届中医学术会议论文汇编, 1979: 201
27. 温州市医药科学研究所, 慢性气管炎血浆内环核苷酸水平与中医脏腑分型关系的初步报告, 浙江中医杂志, 1981; 16（1）: 2
28. 广西中医学院中医理论研究室.肺气虚病人血清α1—抗胰蛋白水平的初步观察, 广西中医药, 1981; （4）: 41
29. 刘中杰. 肺气虚证患者体液免疫变化的研究, 中国医药学报, 1994, (4): 28
30. 王会仍等.肺气虚与慢性阻塞性肺病关系及其本质的研究, 中国医药学报, 1992, 7（4）: 62
31. 李平.40 例肺气虚患者血清干扰素活性观察, 安徽中医学院学报 , 1991, 10(1): 43
32. 赵江云等.肺气虚、肺气阴两虚患者 T 淋巴细胞亚群的观察, 安徽中医学院学报, 1993, 12（1）: 49

33. 陆桂祥等.百年乐对肺气虚病人免疫功能及血锌浓度的影响, 广西中医药, 1993, 16（2）: 47
34. 郭孝月等.小儿肺脾气虚咳嗽微观研究, 山东中医学院学报, 1994, 18（2）: 102.
35. 王元勋等.肺气虚证的实验研究—免疫功能状态的研究 I, 甘肃中医学院学报, 1993, 10（3）: 52.
36. 宋卫东.肺气虚患者支气管及肺泡灌洗液中细胞成分的变化, 安徽中医学院学报, 1993, 12（4）: 43.
37. 刘中本等.肺气虚患者体液免疫变化的研究, 中国医药学报, 1994, 9（4）: 28.
38. 郭孝月等.保肺片治疗小儿脾肺气虚型咳嗽的临床研究, 山东中医学院学报, 1994, 18（6）: 396.
39. 马融等.抗感至宝口服液防治小儿反复呼吸道感染的临床研究, 中国中西医结合杂志, 1994, 14（10）: 586.
40. 蔡丽芬.肺气虚证与免疫球蛋白 G 和白细胞计数相关性的临床观察, 湖北中医杂志, 1995, 17（4）: 13
41. 钱朝余等.补肺定喘丸对肺虚型喘缓解期疗效观察, 新中医, 1996, 28（1）: 26.
42. 许得盛.益气化痰、益气健脾、化痰法治疗慢性支气管炎的疗效比较, 上海中医药杂志, 1999, （8）: 12
43. 徐小玉等.益气免疫冲剂治疗气虚证慢性阻塞性肺病 72 例观察, 中国中西医结合杂志, 1996, 16（2）: 81
44. 李平等.肺气虚证与红细胞 SOD 活性、变形能力及 C3b 受体关系的研究, 实用中西医结合杂志, 1996, 9（4）: 201.
45. 赵湘等.小剂量灭活卡介苗对慢性阻塞性肺病肺气虚患者细胞免疫功能影响, 中国中西医结合杂志, 1996, 16（7）: 408.
46. 宋卫东等.肺泡巨噬细胞对肺气虚证局部神经 内分泌 免疫系统功能影响, 中国中医基础医学杂志, 1997, 3（4）: 31
47. 王宪富等.康莱特对肺癌切除术后肺气虚免疫功能低下患者的临床观察, 中国中西医结合杂志, 1998, 18（7）: 431
48. 徐锡鸿等.肺气虚证患者的免疫功能探析, 中医药研究, 1999, 15（3）: 37.
49. 杨牧祥等.对“肺气虚证”大鼠肺组织及支气管 NOS 的检测, 中医杂志, 1999, 40（2）: 107.

50. 徐锡鸣等.肺气虚证患者支气管黏膜超微结构观察, 中医杂志, 1999, 40（9）: 556.
51. 朴胜夫等.肺心病病人自由基代谢的研究, 中华结核和呼吸杂志, 1992, 15（4）: 214.
52. 程惠娟等.肺气虚证患者血浆纤维结合素及血气分析的初步观察, 甘肃中医学院学报, 1 995, 12（1）: 13.
53. 李泽庚等.肺气虚证与自由基代谢初探—附 102 例资料, 辽宁中医杂志, 1995, 22（5）, 207.
54. 宋卫东等, 肺气虚证肺泡巨噬细胞氧自由基代谢特点, 中国中医基础医学杂志, 1996 , (1): 44
55. 赵江云等.支气管肺灌洗液中 SOD 和 LPO 与肺气虚证的关系, 中国中西医结合杂志, 1996, 16（7）, 405
56. 赵世芬等.益气定喘汤对哮喘豚鼠肺泡巨噬细胞抗氧化能力的影响, 中国中医基础医学杂志, 2000, 6（2）, 31.
57. 许涛等.心钠素在肺气虚证诊断中的意义, 甘肃中医学院学报, 2000, l7（4）: 6.
58. 李君等.内皮素与肺气虚证关系的实验研究, 中医杂志, 2000, 41（10）: 618.
59. 同 27.
60. 古传琼, 慢性支气管炎中西医结合分型血浆 cAMP 和 cGMP 测定的初步观察, 天津医药, 1982, (2): 117
61. 同 28.
62. 林文森等.鼻腔分泌物环核苷酸含量与慢性支气管炎辨证分型的关系, 浙江中医杂志, 1982, 17(11): 522
63. 同 19.
64. 汪慰寒.心纳素在心肺气虚诊断中的意义, 中西医结合杂志, 1988; 8（6）: 521
65. 齐幼龄等.88 例肺气虚病人血浆肾素、血管紧张素□及醛固酮的测定, 广西中医药, 1991, 14(2): 93
66. 江明等.慢支肺脾肾虚证型与血环核苷酸 cAMP 和 CGMP 关系的探讨, 福建中医学院学报, 1995, 5（1）: 16.
67. 宋卫东等.肺泡巨细胞内 cAMP 和 cGMP 与肺气虚证的关系, 中国医药学报, 1995, 10（1）: 21.

68. 赵江云等.肺气虚证局部内分泌功能紊乱对肺泡巨噬细胞影响, 中国中医基础医学杂志, 1996, 2（2）: 16.
69. 钱宝庆. 肺心 2 号方对 31 例肺心病肺肾气虚型者头发中某些微量元素的影响及疗效观察, 浙江中医学院学报, 1990, (2): 27
70. 谭茹.小儿反复呼吸道感染肺气虚证与微量元素的研究, 辽宁中医杂志, 1991, 18(7): 8
71. 陆桂祥等.百年乐对肺气虚病人免疫功能及血锌浓度的影响, 广西中医药, 1993, 16（2）: 47
72. 全润芍等.慢阻肺病人肺气虚证治疗前后微量元素含量的改变—附 60 例分析, 中医研究, 1994, 7（2）: 16.
73. 周庆伟.对肺气虚患者微量元素及肺功能的临床观察, 中国医药学报, 1996, 11（6）: 25.
74. 耿宏伟.中药对肺气虚患者微量元素及肺功能的影响, 中国中医药信息杂志, 2000, 7（10）: 41.
75. 赵勤萍等.慢性支气管肺炎肺气虚证 6 种微量元素变化规律研究, 中医杂志, 1999, 40（1）: 44.
76. 同 28.
77. 徐锡鸿等.肺气虚证患者支气管黏膜超微结构观察, 中医杂志, 1999, 40（9）: 556.
78. 杨牧祥等.实验性“肺气虚证”肺组织病理研究, 河北医科大学学报, 1996, 17（6）: 344.
79. 刘素蓉.阴虚阳虚证与血液流变学研究, 中国医药学报, 1989, 4(2): 12
80. 张凤瑞等.肺阴虚实质研究进展, 吉林中医药, 1994, (5): 40
81. 邵长荣.养阴法治疗阴虚型肺结核及其对细胞免疫的观察, 上海中医药杂志, 1980, (2): 19
82. 邵长荣.肺结核阴虚证与细胞介导的细胞毒性试验, 辽宁中医杂志, 1986, (1): 43
83. 何雄等.肺阴虚型浸润型肺结核患者的 NK 细胞活性缺陷, 中医药学报, 1991, (5): 47
84. 南征等.中医肺阴虚证免疫机能的研究, 吉林中医药, 1990, (5): 34
85. 宓雅珠等.肺阴虚证 T-淋巴细胞亚群状态的初步研究, 辽宁中医杂志 1999, 26（5）: 208

86. 王正昌等.肺癌患者三种虚证类型的治疗生存期与血浆环核苷酸水平的关系, 中西医结合杂志, 1984, 4(l): 23
87. 马贵同.气阴两虚病人铜、锌、铁微量元素变化的初步观察, 上海中医药杂志, 1985, (8): 2
88. 邱保国等.虚证病人头发五种微量元素分析, 中医杂志, 1985, 26(1): 59
89. 夏以琳等.呼吸道反复感染儿童头发微量元素分析, 辽宁中医杂志, 1991, 18(7): 6
90. 戴豪良等.肺肾阴虚证患者头发中微量元素的初步观察, 中医研究, 1990, 3(2): 21
91. 杨德诚等.呼吸系统疾病肺阴虚证人发 15 种元素值的多元逐步分析, 吉林中医药, 1994, (1): 44

Chinese Books

《黄帝内经•素问》. 北京: 人民卫生出版社, 1965.
《灵枢经》. 北京: 人民卫生出版社, 1965.

四画

方隅.《医林绳墨》.上海: 商务印书馆, 1957.
王叔和.《脉经》. 北京: 人民卫生出版社, 1956.
王肯堂.《证治准绳》.上海: 上海卫生出版社, 1958.
王焘.《外台秘要》.北京: 人民卫生出版社, 1955.
王怀隐.《太平圣惠方》. 北京: 人民卫生出版社, 1958.
王纶.《明医杂著》.江苏: 科学技术出版社, 1985.
王孟英.《温热经纬》.北京: 人民卫生出版社, 1956.
王清任.《医林改错》.上海: 上海科学技术出版社, 1966.
王琦.《中医藏象学》.北京: 人民卫生出版社, 1997.
王新华.《中医药高级丛书中医基础理论》. 北京: 人民卫生出版社, 2001.
尤在泾.《金匮要略心典》.上海: 上海卫生出版社, 1975.
尤在泾.《金匮翼》. 上海: 上海卫生出版社, 1957.
丹波元坚.《杂病广要》. 北京: 人民卫生出版社, 1958.

五画

冯楚瞻.《冯氏锦囊秘录》. 北京: 人民卫生出版社, 1996.
叶天士.《临证指南医案》.上海: 上海人民出版社, 1976.

卢和.《丹溪纂要》.见金元四大家医学全书, 天津: 天津科学技术出版社, 1983.
北山友松子（日）.《医方考绳愆》.天津: 天津市新华书店古旧书门市部, 1980.

六画

刘完素.《素问玄机原病式》.北京: 人民卫生出版社, 1956.
刘完素.《素问病机气宜保命集》.北京: 人民卫生出版社, 1959.
刘松峰.《松峰说疫》. 北京: 人民卫生出版社, 1987.
江涵暾.《笔花医镜》.上海: 上海科学技术出版社, 1958.
许浚等.《东医宝鉴》. 北京: 人民卫生出版社, 1955.
华佗.《中藏经》.北京: 人民卫生出版社, 1990.朱震亨.《丹溪心法》.上海: 上海科学技术出版社, 1959.
朱震亨.《脉因证治》.上海: 上海科学技术出版社, 1958.
危亦林.《世医得效方》.北京: 人民卫生出版社, 1990.
孙思邈.《千金要方》.北京: 人民卫生出版社, 1955.
孙思邈.《千金翼方》.北京: 人民卫生出版社, 1955.

七画

汪绮石.《理虚元鉴》. 北京: 人民卫生出版社, 1988.
汪讱庵.《医方集解》. 上海: 上海科学技术出版社, 1959.
沈金鳌.《杂病源流犀烛》.上海: 上海科学技术出版社, 1962.
沈朗仲.《病机汇论》. 北京: 人民卫生出版社, 1996.
沈青芝.《喉科集腋》.北京: 中国古籍出版社, 1982.
李中梓.《医宗必读》.上海: 上海卫生出版社, 1957.
李用粹.《证治汇补》.上海: 上海科学技术出版社, 1956.
李东垣.《内外伤辨惑论》.北京: 人民卫生出版社, 1959.
李东垣.《脾胃论》. 北京: 人民卫生出版社, 1957.
李东垣.《东垣十书》.千顷堂石印本, 清光绪 33 年（1907）
李梴.《医学入门》. 北京: 中国中医药出版社, 1999.
李乃季等.《永类钤方》.北京: 北京大学影印本
李冠仙.《知医必辨》. 江苏: 科学技术出版社, 1984.
杨士瀛.《仁斋直指附遗方论》.上海: 上海古籍出版社, 1991.
杨乘六.《医宗己任编》. 上海: 上海卫生出版社, 1958.
严用和.《济生方》.北京: 人民卫生出版社, 1956.
吴坤安.《伤寒指掌》.上海: 上海科学技术出版社, 1959.
吴鹤皋.《医方考》.北京: 人民卫生出版社, 1990.
吴澄.《不居集》. 北京: 人民卫生出版社, 1996.
吴鞠通.《温病条辨》.北京: 人民卫生出版社, 1957.

吴谦等.《医宗金鉴》.北京: 人民卫生出版社, 1963.
余根初.《重订通俗伤寒论》. 上海: 上海科学技术出版社, 1959.
何梦瑶.《医碥》.上海: 上海科学技术出版社, 1982.
张三锡.《治法汇》.见医学六要, 明崇祯十七年甲申复印本
张子和.《儒门事亲》. 上海: 上海科学技术出版社, 1959.
张介宾.《景岳全书》.北京: 人民卫生出版社, 1990.
张介宾.《类经》.北京: 人民卫生出版社, 1957.
张介宾.《类经附翼》.北京: 人民卫生出版社, 1957.
张仲景.《伤寒论》.北京: 人民卫生出版社, 1991.
张仲景.《金匮要略》.北京: 人民卫生出版社, 1991.
张路玉.《张氏医通》.上海: 上海科学技术出版社, 1963.
张锡纯.《医学衷中参西录》.河北人民出版社, 1977.
陈言.《三因极一病证方论》. 北京: 人民卫生出版社, 1957.
陈士铎.《辨证录》.北京: 人民卫生出版社, 1965.
陈士铎.《石室秘录》.北京: 中国中医药出版社, 1991
陈自民.《妇人良方》.上海: 上海卫生出版社, 1956.
陈师文.《太平惠民和剂局方》.北京: 人民卫生出版社, 1985.
陈梦雷.《图书集成医部全录》. 北京: 人民卫生出版社, 1963.

八画

金礼蒙.《医方类聚》.北京: 人民卫生出版社, 1981.
郑钦安.《医理真传》.成都: 巴蜀书社, 1988.
林佩琴.《类证治裁》.上海: 上海科学技术出版社, 1959.
罗天益.《卫生宝鉴》. 北京: 人民卫生出版社, 1963.
罗国纲.《罗氏会约医镜》.北京: 人民卫生出版社, 1965.
周学海.《读医笔记》.南京: 江苏科学技术出版社, 1983.
周慎斋.《慎斋遗书》. 上海: 上海科学技术出版社, 1959.

九画

赵佶.《圣济总录》.北京: 人民卫生出版社, 1962.
赵献可.《医贯》..北京: 人民卫生出版社, 1959.
赵绍琴等.《温病纵横》. 北京: 人民卫生出版社, 1982.
皇甫中.《明医指掌》. 北京: 人民卫生出版社, 1982.
贵阳中医学院.《方剂学》.贵阳: 贵州人民出版社, 1989.

十画

徐仁斋.《重订通俗伤寒论》.杭州: 新医书局出版社, 1956.
唐宗海.《血证论》. 北京: 人民卫生出版社, 1990.
唐宗海.《金匮要略浅注补正》.上海: 上海大达图书供应社, 1935.

顾松园.《顾松园医镜》. 郑州: 河南人民卫生出版社, 1961.
秦景明.《症因脉治》.上海: 上海科学技术出版社, 1990.
秦越人.《难经》.北京: 人民卫生出版社, 1991.
钱仲阳.《小儿药证直诀》.北京: 人民卫生出版社, 1955.
钱潢.《伤寒溯源集》. 上海: 上海卫生出版社, 1957
徐春甫.《古今医统大全》.南京: 南京中医学院影印, 1984.
载原礼.《证治要诀》. 上海: 上海商务印书馆, 1955.

十一画

章潢.《图书编》.见四库全书 127 卷子部类书类.
黄元御.《四圣心源》.北京: 中国医药出版社, 1996
龚云林.《寿世保元》.上海: 上海科学技术出版社, 1959.
龚信.《古今医鉴》.上海: , 1997.
崔家彦.《脉诀》.见古今医统正脉全书, 明万历 29 年吴勉学校刻本（1601）
巢元方.《诸病源候论》. 北京: 人民卫生出版社, 1955.

十二画

董宿.《奇效良方》.上海: 商务书印馆, 1956.
葛洪.《肘后方》.北京: 人民卫生出版社, 1957.
程文囿.《医述》.合肥: 安徽科学技术出版社, 1983.
程国彭.《医学心悟》.北京: 人民卫生出版社, 1963.

十三画

雷丰.《时病论》. 北京: 人民卫生出版社, 1972.
喻嘉言.《医门法律》. 上海: 上海科学技术出版社, 1963
蒲辅周.《蒲辅周医疗经验》.北京: 人民卫生出版社, 1976.

Index

—B—

—F—

—G—

—H—

—I—

—J—

—M—

—N—

—O—

—P—

—T—

—U—

FOUNDATION TEXTS FROM PARADIGM PUBLICATIONS

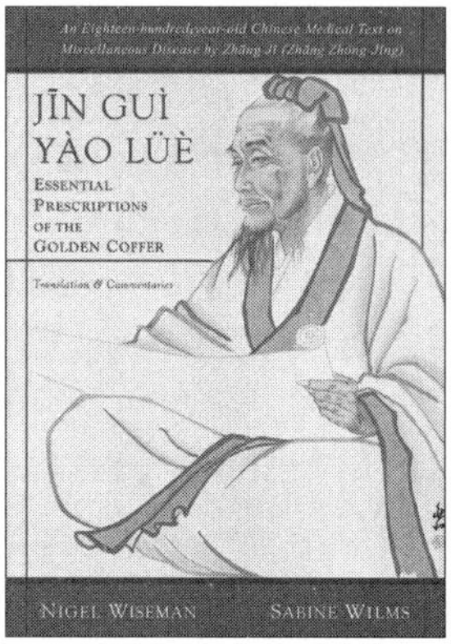

JĪN GUÌ YÀO LÜÈ
ESSENTIAL PRESCRIPTIONS OF THE GOLDEN COFFER
Zháng Zhòng-Jǐng
Translated by Nigel Wiseman and Sabine Wilms
Clothbound, 650 pp, 2011

SHĀNG HÁN LÙN
ON COLD DAMAGE
Zháng Zhòng-Jǐng
Translated by Craig Mitchell and Nigel Wiseman
Clothbound, 746 pp, 1999

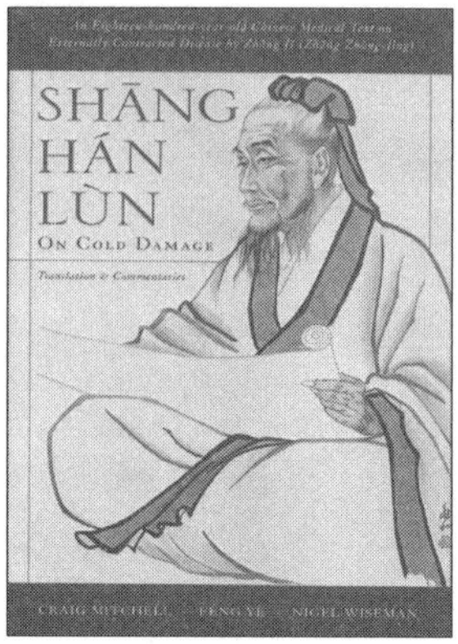

The ***Shāng Hán Lùn (On Cold Damage)*** has been a primary resource for herbal medical theory and practical therapy in China for nearly two millenia. Its author, Zháng Zhòng-Jǐng, is revered as the "Chinese Hippocrates," highlighting the depth and breadth of his contribution to traditional Chinese medicinal therapy. This edition features the Chinese text, Pinyin transliteration, and an English translation of the entire Song Dynasty text, the content and textual order most used in Asia. Just as in Chinese language editions, it is fully supplemented with notes and commentaries. The notes describe the clinical symptoms Zháng Zhòng-Jǐng associated with the Chinese terms. Extensive commentaries further enhance the text's clinical utility by explaining the theoretical and practical foundations behind the lines of text. Because entire bodies of theory and practice can be associated with the terms and expressions used in canonical works like the *Shāng Hán Lùn*, commentaries a rich source of knowledge acquisition. The introductory matter explains the background of the text, the conceptual structure of its contents, and the problems of exegesis. The appendices are designed to assist those studying Chinese and the glossary and the full Pinyin-English index make this an easily accessed reference.

The ***Jīn Guì Yào Lüè (Essential Prescriptions of the Golden Coffer),*** like its sister volume the *Shāng Hán Lùn (On Cold Damage)*, is a gem reconstituted from fragments of a lost text called the *Shāng Hán Zá Bìng Lùn (On Cold Damage and Miscellaneous Diseases),* written by indisputably the most brilliant medical mind China ever produced, the Han Dynasty physician Zháng Zhòng-Jǐng. Exerting an influence on the development of Chinese medicine unmatched by any other medical scholar, Zháng integrated the then relatively new theories of systematic correspondence from the *Nèijīng* and *Nànjīng* with his already vast practical knowledge in the use of medicinals. Such was his brilliance that it was not fully recognized by Chinese physicians until centuries later in the Sòng Dynasty, when Zháng's combination of theory and practice became the mainstream in Chinese medicine that survived centuries of scrutiny from successive generations of medical scholars and buttressed traditional medicine against the challenge of Western in the 20th century. Combining theoretic etiologies with detailed diagnosis and skillfully devised treatments, Zháng's work has bequeathed a significant influence on traditional medicine in China for nearly 2,000 years. One-third of the most commonly used formulas in Chinese medical practice today were devised by Zháng Zhòng-Jǐng. The *Jīn Guì Yào Lüè* covers diseases other than external contractions dealt with in the *Shāng Hán Lùn*, including lung diseases, water swelling, dissipation-thirst, impediment (*bì*), summerheat stroke, mounting diseases, and gynecological diseases, to name just a few. The first chapter explains the etiology of disease and treatment principles, while the last discusses food prohibitions.